Don't let high cholesterol fool you.

Sure, it's virtually symptom-free. But high cholesterol is a major contributor to heart disease, the leading cause of death in the United States. The good news is it is very treatable—and you may not need medication. Often, lifestyle changes alone are enough.

Just ask any of the 100 women and men whose stories appear here. Some had family histories of heart disease and wanted to avoid the same fate. Others stood on the brink of heart attack, or had surgery to repair the damage high cholesterol had done. Walking helped Bonnie Luft shave 115 points from her total cholesterol. Bill Israel started eating oatmeal for breakfast and his cholesterol plummeted over 80 points. For Joanna Pucel, who had a coronary bypass at age thirty-seven, daily relaxation breaks help lower her "bad" LDL cholesterol 131 points and raise her "good" HDL cholesterol 43 points.

Their stories, and ninety-seven others, are proof positive that a healthy cholesterol profile is within reach. And their Winning Actions have been reviewed by experts, so you can use them with confidence. In short, *Win the Cholesterol War* gives you everything you need to achieve healthy cholesterol levels.

WIN THE CHOLESTEROL WAR

100 REAL-LIFE

SECRETS TO

TRIMMING POINTS (AND POUNDS)

Holly McCord, R.D.
nutrition editor, *Prevention*® magazine

BERKLEY BOOKS, NEW YORK

WIN THE CHOLESTEROL WAR

A Berkley Book / published by arrangement with Rodale Inc.

NOTE: Every effort has been made to ensure that the information contained in this book is complete and accurate. However, neither the publisher nor the author is engaged in rendering professional advice or services to the individual reader. The ideas, procedures, and suggestions contained in this book are not intended as a substitute for consulting with your physician. All matters regarding your health require medical supervision. Neither the author nor the publisher shall be liable or responsible for any loss, injury, or damage allegedly arising from any information or suggestion in this book. The opinions expressed in this book represent the personal views of the author and not of the publisher.

PRINTING HISTORY
Rodale hardcover edition / October 2001
Berkley edition / January 2003

Win the Fat War is a trademark and *Prevention* is a registered trademark of Rodale Inc.

Visit our website at
www.penguinputnam.com

ISBN: 0-425-18819-1

BERKLEY®
Berkley Books are published by The Berkley Publishing Group, a division of Penguin Putnam Inc., 375 Hudson Street, New York, New York 10014.
BERKLEY and the "B" design
are trademarks belonging to Penguin Putnam Inc.

PRINTED IN THE UNITED STATES OF AMERICA

10 9 8 7 6 5 4 3 2

CONTENTS

✦ ✦ ✦

ACKNOWLEDGMENTS

✦ ✦ ✦

This book would not exist were it not for the extraordinary talent and sheer hard work of my colleagues in the Rodale Women's Health Group. For their efforts, my heartfelt thanks go to Catherine Cassidy, Tami Booth, Susan Berg, Madeleine Adams, Jane Sherman, Sandi Lloyd, Shea Zukowski, Jennifer Goldsmith, Molly Brown, Lucille Uhlman, Lori Davis, Barbara Thomas-Fexa, Jan McLeod, Josh Popichak, Karen Jacob, Rebecca Theodore, Liz Price, Carrie Havranek, Darlene Schneck, Carol Angstadt, Christina Gaugler, Bethany Bodder, Marilyn Hauptly, Julie Kehs Minnix, Jodi Schaffer, Amy Rhodes, Leslie Schneider, Shannon Gallagher, Dana Bacher, Lorraine Rodriguez, Lisa Dolin, Tawan Smith, Cindy Ratzlaff, and Mary Lengle.

Thanks, too, to Jean Rogers, Laura Catalano, Linda Formichelli, W. Eric Martin, Lynn Reynolds Parks, and Winnie Yu for their editorial contributions, and to Robert S. Rosenson, M.D., director of the preventive cardiology center at Northwestern University Medical School in Chicago, for his invaluable expert review of the Winning Actions that appear throughout the book.

Of course, I'm extraordinarily grateful to the 100 men and women who graciously volunteered to share their stories for the book. Their willingness to invite us into their lives so that we might benefit from their experiences has touched me deeply.

A number of these people came to us through Mended Hearts, a support group for heart disease patients and their families. To learn more about the organization's services, visit www.mendedhearts.org or call (800) AHA-USA1 (800-242-8721) and ask for Mended Hearts support.

INTRODUCTION

✦ ✦ ✦

YES, YOU CAN WIN THE
CHOLESTEROL WAR!

I admit, I'm very lucky. I've never had to contend with high cholesterol. Mine has always stayed right about where it should be. But I know plenty of people who struggle with cholesterol problems. As nutrition editor for *Prevention* magazine, I regularly hear from readers who want to know what they can do, nutrition-wise, to get their numbers to healthier levels.

That's why I jumped at the chance to do this book. It's going to help spread the word that high cholesterol is not just controllable but curable.

Make no mistake: High cholesterol is serious business. Even though you can't feel it, it's doing its dirty work inside your arteries, building up plaques that can eventually block bloodflow to your heart or brain and trigger a heart attack or stroke.

According to the American Heart Association, high cholesterol affects more than 100 million Americans. Many of them probably don't know it because they're not getting their cholesterol checked as often as they should. And even those who have been diagnosed may not be managing their cholesterol effectively because they're not sure what to do.

I suspect you've picked up this book because you're in this situation yourself. Perhaps you've tried following your doctor's advice to "eat right and exercise regularly," but you're having trouble sticking with it. Or maybe you've been given a prescription for a cholesterol-lowering medication, but you don't like the idea of taking pills for the rest of your life. (A word of caution, however: If you are taking any medicine, you should not stop without talking to your doctor. He knows your medical history better than anyone and can help plan the best course of treatment for you.)

What matters most is that you've made a decision to change your cholesterol profile for the better. In that fact alone, you have a great deal in common with the men and women interviewed for this book. But that's not the only aspect of their stories that should strike a familiar chord. In their struggles to resist a favorite food that's packed with saturated fat, to slip into their workout clothes instead of sliding onto the sofa, to alter the course of their family history by beating the odds against heart disease, you just may see a part of yourself.

That's why their stories feel so compelling and inspirational. Each time I read about their experiences, I'm blown away by the odds they've beaten. Some of these people shouldn't be alive today; even their doctors said so. Yet they're not just surviving but thriving—living proof that the cholesterol war can be won, no matter where you are in the battle.

In the course of interviewing men and women for this book, we asked them to identify the one tip or technique that they feel made the biggest difference in bringing their cholesterol under control. These Winning Actions appear at the end of the respective personal profiles. While the strategies have been shown to work, at least anecdotally, we went the extra step of putting them through medical review to ensure that they're safe and responsible.

To help you navigate the book, the personal profiles are organized into four sections. "Eat Well to Win," beginning on page 40, focuses on dietary changes—perhaps the most important and most challenging aspect of any cholesterol treatment plan. "Shape Up Your Cholesterol Profile" (page 100) offers advice on building more physical activity into your day. If you want to know more about nondrug remedies for high cholesterol, the stories in "Get the Numbers You Want Naturally" (page 151) may have the information you're looking for. In "Stay on Track for Success" (page 189), you'll find motivational strategies that can help you stick with whatever course of treatment you choose.

I recommend reading through the three introductory chapters first. They'll tell you more about cholesterol—why we need it, why we end up with too much of it, and how to interpret your numbers—and give you a brief overview of some of the most popular treatments. Also included are the Ten Commandments of Cholesterol Control, which can provide a solid foundation for any cholesterol treatment plan.

Armed with this knowledge, you're set to pick and choose from the 100 Winning Actions that appear in the rest of the book. Try them one at a time and give each an opportunity to work. If it doesn't produce the results you expect, move on to something else.

One final note: Throughout this book, we've based our evaluations of individual cholesterol readings on the guidelines established by the American Heart Association. These guidelines have been updated to match the recommendations released in May 2001 by the National Cholesterol Education Program, a branch of the National Heart, Lung, and Blood

Institute. They'll help you determine where your cholesterol stands and where it ought to be in order to reduce your heart disease risk.

You hold the secrets of successful cholesterol control in your hands—literally. Take action now, and enjoy healthy cholesterol for life!

THE TEN COMMANDMENTS
OF CHOLESTEROL CONTROL

✦ ✦ ✦

You've been diagnosed with high cholesterol. Now what? It's a perfectly valid question, the same one facing millions of Americans at this very moment. Your doctor has probably recommended dietary changes, perhaps more exercise, maybe even medication. But you know you can do more. You're just not sure what, or when, or how.

That's why we've created the Ten Commandments of Cholesterol Control. They're the basic steps anyone can follow, no matter what their current cholesterol profile, to get the numbers they want.

Some of the commandments may seem more important to you than others, depending on your current health status. For now, feel free to focus on those most relevant to your situation. You can return to the others later; at the very least, they'll help you stay informed and inspired as you wage your own cholesterol war.

Just remember that by adopting all ten commandments, you establish a solid foundation for lifelong cholesterol control. They'll support whatever treatment plan you ultimately choose to follow. There's no better time to get started than now!

1. Know Where You Stand

You've heard the old saying about no news being good news? Well, it doesn't apply to cholesterol. Getting it checked on a regular basis is essential to your long-term good health. After all, high cholesterol has been linked to cardiovascular disease, the number one cause of death in the United States. In fact, according to the American Heart Association, people who have a total cholesterol of 240 mg/dL (milligrams per deciliter) are *twice* as likely to experience a heart attack as people who have a cholesterol level of 200 mg/dL. Knowing your level, and tracking it as you begin treatment, just makes sense.

We'll discuss cholesterol screening in detail in the next chapter. In a nutshell, all adults age 20 and over should have their cholesterol checked at least once every 5 years as recommended by the National Heart, Lung, and Blood Institute of the National Institutes of Health. You may require more frequent screening if you have certain risk factors for heart disease or if your test results are cause for concern.

Generally, doctors like to see total cholesterol below 200 mg/dL, with LDL (bad cholesterol) below 130—the high end of the "near-optimal" range—and HDL (good cholesterol) above 40. If your test results aren't consistent with these levels, your doctor may recommend a retest. If they're still not where they should be, your doctor may want to discuss treatment options.

The truly good news is that in many cases, cholesterol is easily managed, even without medication. But you need to know your starting point, and you need to monitor your progress toward healthy levels. Even for those whose cholesterol is within the range considered normal, knocking a few points off their readings can slow fatty buildup in the arteries and possibly reduce any buildup that's already there. The bottom line: In the pursuit of cholesterol control, knowing your numbers is an absolute necessity.

2. Learn All You Can

Once you've been diagnosed with high cholesterol, your instinct may be to jump right into whatever treatment plan your doctor recommends. Unless your cholesterol has gone through the roof, which may require immediate intervention, you're better off taking time to think through your situation and your treatment options. By exercising some control upfront, you're more likely to develop a cholesterol management plan you can truly live with.

Perhaps a good place to begin is with an assessment of your personal risk factors for heart disease beyond high cholesterol. Which ones are within your control? For example, you may not be able to change your age, gender, or family history. But you can improve your eating habits, get more exercise, and quit smoking. These are the sorts of lifestyle changes that should become part of your cholesterol management plan, no matter what other treatments you may choose.

Likewise, you'll want to learn as much as you can about cholesterol itself. As the next chapter explains, your body needs cholesterol to perform certain vital functions. In fact, lowering one type of cholesterol, HDL, can be bad for your heart. What's more, while many foods contain dietary cholesterol, most of the blame for elevated cholesterol levels rests squarely on the shoulders of saturated fat.

Of course, you'll also want to educate yourself about the available treatment options. As you'll discover in Treatments Your Heart Will Love, on page 24, conventional medicine has much to offer to people with high cholesterol—but so do alternative therapies. Indeed, the choices can seem overwhelming. Before you settle on a specific treatment or combination of treatments (in consultation with your doctor), you should know whether it's effective and safe and how soon you can expect to see results.

This book will give you a solid overview of cholesterol and its potential treatments. For additional information, consider checking out the American Heart Association Web site located at www.americanheart.org or the National Heart, Lung, and Blood Institute's site at www.nhlbi.nih.gov. Another good resource: *Prevention* magazine's Web site at www.prevention.com.

3. Get Rid of Those Extra Pounds

If you weigh more than you should, slimming down may produce a significant drop in your cholesterol level. Research suggests that being overweight disrupts the normal metabolism of dietary fat. So even though you may be eating less fat, you may not see a difference in your cholesterol profile until you unload the excess pounds.

In fact, shedding just 5 to 10 pounds may be enough to improve your cholesterol level. Just don't go the crash-dieting route. A slow but steady loss of ½ to 1 pound a week is healthiest and easiest to maintain. Since 1 pound equals 3,500 calories, you could meet the pound-per-week rate by eating 500 fewer calories per day, burning 500 more calories per day through exercise, or—the best option—a combination of the two.

Findings from the landmark Framingham Heart Study confirm that such modest weight loss is worth the effort, for reasons beyond cholesterol control. According to the study, taking off—and keeping off—just 1 to 2 pounds a year may reduce your risk of high blood pressure by 25 percent and your risk of diabetes by 35 percent.

Incidentally, many of the lifestyle strategies that help rein in unruly cholesterol can also take off unwanted pounds, and vice versa. If you're significantly overweight, be sure to consult your doctor before embarking on any weight-loss program.

4. Lace Up Your Walking Shoes

Whether your goal is to lower your cholesterol, shed some extra pounds, or both, regular exercise can help you get there. We're not talking about high-intensity workouts, either, though boosting your intensity can elevate HDL cholesterol. Walking and other, more moderate physical activities are good for your heart, too.

In fact, one study suggests that walks of any duration may help reduce heart disease risk. For the study, British researchers recruited 56 sedentary people between ages 40 and 66, then divided them into three groups. One group took a long, 20- to 40-minute walk each day; another group walked for 10 to 15 minutes twice a day; and the third group took 5- to 10-minute walks three times a day.

Over the 18 weeks of the study, the once-a-day walkers saw their LDL cholesterol drop by 8.3 percent; the twice-a-day walkers by 5.8 percent. The researchers concluded that walks of any length can be beneficial, as long as they're done at a moderate intensity—that is, a brisk pace at which you can still carry on a conversation.

We mention walking because it's the most convenient form of physical activity. But really, any form of aerobic exercise—running, bicycling, swimming, whatever gets your heart pumping—can help lower heart disease risk. Whichever activity (or activities) you choose, just make sure you're doing it for 30 minutes at least 5 days a week.

If you've been relatively inactive, check with your doctor before launching any exercise regimen. Your doctor may be able to help you choose an activity that suits your current fitness level.

5. Become Acquainted with the Good Fats

When you were diagnosed with high cholesterol, your doctor likely advised you to reduce your fat intake. In general, cutting your dietary fat will lower cholesterol. But as with any rule, this one has exceptions. Evidence suggests that eating more of some fats and less of others is better than simply cutting way back on all fats.

Peanut butter, avocados, olive and canola oils, and most nuts are mostly monounsaturated fat. Research has shown that monounsaturated fat can help lower LDL and triglycerides (another type of blood fat) while raising HDL. It's a much healthier choice than saturated fat, found primarily in animal products—meats, butter, full-fat milk and cheese. Saturated fat can elevate your cholesterol level more than anything else you might eat.

Also included in the good fats category are the omega-3 fatty acids, found in abundance in fish such as mackerel, albacore tuna, and salmon. The omega-3's appear to lower levels of VLDL (very low density lipoprotein) and triglycerides. Studies have shown that when people cut back on saturated fat and consumed more fish oil, their LDL dropped. The American Heart Association recommends eating at least 2 servings of baked or grilled fish a week.

That said, omega-3's are not a magic bullet. When study participants consumed more fish oil without altering their saturated fat intake, their LDL levels stayed the same or increased. In order to reap the cholesterol-cutting benefits of omega-3's, you need to limit your saturated fat consumption. Remember, too, that eating foods low in total fat can help restrict saturated fat.

6. Discover Fiber's Cholesterol-Cutting Capacity

It's no secret that vegetarians have lower cholesterol levels and lower heart disease rates than meat-eaters. That's in part because vegetarians consume so much fiber, which is found exclusively in plant foods—fruits, vegetables, whole grains, and beans.

Fiber comes in two forms: soluble and insoluble. The soluble kind appears to pack the greatest cholesterol-lowering punch. Research has shown that consuming about 15 grams of soluble fiber a day can lower LDL cholesterol by 5 to 10 percent. It works by binding with cholesterol-containing bile acids in the intestines and escorting them out of the body.

A specific kind of soluble fiber, pectin, not only lowers cholesterol but also helps curb overeating by slowing the digestive process. Munch on apples and other pectin-rich fruits, and you're likely to eat less, lose weight, *and* rein in your cholesterol.

Coincidentally, foods high in fiber tend to be low in saturated fat and cholesterol, as well as calories. Just make sure you don't top your fiber-rich whole grain toast with a huge dollop of butter.

7. Take a Good Multivitamin

Even if you're getting more good fats, avoiding bad fats, and filling up on fiber, your diet may have some nutritional gaps. A multivitamin/mineral supplement can help cover your nutritional bases and possibly lower your risk for heart disease and stroke.

Look for a multi that delivers 400 micrograms of folic acid, 2 milligrams of vitamin B_6, and 6 micrograms of vitamin B_{12}, advises Robert Rosenson, M.D., director of the preventive cardiology center at Northwestern University

Medical School in Chicago. In studies, all three of these B vitamins have played important roles in protecting heart health.

In a Harvard study involving 80,000 nurses, for example, those with the highest intakes of folic acid were 31 percent less likely to develop heart disease. Folic acid works by decreasing blood levels of homocysteine, an amino acid that's an emerging risk factor for heart disease and stroke. While many foods contain folate (the naturally occurring form of folic acid), including orange juice, kidney beans, broccoli, and spinach, you'll be certain that you're getting the recommended amount by taking a multivitamin.

The same study found that the women who consumed the most vitamin B_6 reduced their risk of heart disease by one-third. Like folic acid, B_6 helps to hold down levels of homocysteine.

In older people, effectively controlling levels of homocysteine may depend on adequate stores of vitamin B_{12}. After age 50, the human body sometimes absorbs less B_{12} from food. According to Johns Hopkins researchers, older people who took a multivitamin containing B_{12} had lower levels of homocysteine.

When you're shopping for a multivitamin, steer clear of those that contain iron. According to Dr. Rosenson, men and postmenopausal women don't need extra iron. Iron stores have been linked with a higher rate of heart attacks and strokes.

8. Explore Your Treatment Options

When you were diagnosed with high cholesterol, you and your doctor probably discussed an appropriate course of treatment. It's important that you continue to work with your doctor and inform him or her of any therapies that you decide to try on your own.

The fact is, both conventional and alternative medicine have a range of cholesterol-combating strategies available.

Which ones you choose depends on your current cholesterol profile, your general health, your lifestyle, even your perspective on treatment. Some people feel perfectly comfortable taking cholesterol-lowering medication, while others do all they can to avoid it.

For people who have advanced heart disease or who've already had a heart attack, conventional therapies such as drugs and surgery are vital, at least at the start of treatment. Later, you and your doctor can discuss lifestyle strategies and alternative therapies that may support your recovery and possibly stop the disease from progressing.

For those with mild to moderately elevated cholesterol, lifestyle strategies and alternative therapies may make drugs and surgery unnecessary, Dr. Rosenson says. These days, many physicians urge patients in the mild-to-moderate category to try controlling their cholesterol through dietary changes and increased physical activity. If those measures alone aren't enough, or if a patient already has coronary heart disease or is at high risk for it, physicians reach for the prescription pad.

Together, you and your doctor can come up with a treatment plan that matches your needs and lifestyle—and that delivers the results you want. In Treatments Your Heart Will Love on page 24, you'll be able to compare several popular conventional and alternative therapies to see which ones might help you rein in your cholesterol.

9. Find Ways to Short-Circuit Stress

To win the cholesterol war, managing stress is as essential as eating healthfully and exercising regularly. When you're tense and anxious, you're more likely to neglect the actions that help lower cholesterol in the first place. After spending 12 hours at the office working frantically to meet a deadline, do you really want to devote another hour to preparing a nutritious meal or walking on a treadmill? Probably not.

What's more, stress and its companion emotions—tension, anxiety, anger, depression—trigger the release of chemicals that constrict arteries, reduce bloodflow to the heart, raise blood pressure, and elevate your heart rate. These changes, in combination with uncontrolled cholesterol, can put you on course for a heart attack.

To block your body's stress response, simply removing yourself from the stressful situation can help. Go for a short walk, practice deep breathing, perform a few simple stretches, meditate—whatever enables you to relax and re-group. You'll feel better, you'll think more clearly, and you'll spare your heart from harm.

No matter how busy you are, set aside a few minutes every day to reflect on yourself and your life. Are you satisfied with the direction you're taking? Are your needs being met? By tuning out the world and turning inward, you remind yourself of what matters most, and you rise above the stressful distractions that undermine your health in so many ways.

While staying in touch with yourself can help you set priorities and adjust your life's course, don't sacrifice family and social relationships. They give your life balance and enable you to cope with stressful situations. Of course, maintaining ties to family and community takes some effort, especially in an era when technology drives our interactions. But it's worth doing, since research has shown that people with fewer social connections are more prone to illness and more likely to die young. On the bright side, the more social connections you have, the better your chances of living longer—free of heart disease and other life-threatening illnesses.

10. Make a Commitment

In the later chapters of this book, you're going to meet 100 men and women who managed to take charge of their cholesterol and achieve their ideal numbers. Many of these people had experienced some life-changing event that forced them to commit themselves to a healthier, cholesterol-lowering lifestyle.

To win the cholesterol war, you must make that same commitment—resolving to take of yourself, to make necessary changes, to live healthfully every day. Your family and your friends can support you, but ultimately, you're the one making the decisions that will have an impact on your health, for better or worse.

You can take control of your cholesterol. The 100 men and women interviewed for this book prove it. Let their experiences inspire you and their Winning Actions motivate you, so you can write your own success story!

CHOLESTEROL 101: THE
FACTS BEYOND THE FIGURES

✦ ✦ ✦

Let's set the record straight: Cholesterol isn't the villain it's been made out to be. The fatlike substance is essential to the formation of cell membranes and some hormones, to name just two of its many biological functions. It circulates in the bloodstream and is present in every single cell.

Our bodies can make all the cholesterol they need. So when we eat foods that contain cholesterol or provide raw material for cholesterol production, we end up with too much. The excess builds up in our arteries, blocks bloodflow, and—left untreated—can set the stage for a heart attack or stroke.

Diet isn't the only risk factor for high cholesterol, though it's certainly a significant one. If you eat a lot of animal products such as meats and dairy products, you're getting a lot of saturated fat, which drives cholesterol levels skyward. You're also more prone to high cholesterol if you're overweight or inactive, or if it runs in your family.

In the purest sense, "high cholesterol" refers to a total cholesterol level that's above a certain number. Actually, your cholesterol profile is a bit more complicated than that, as you'll see in the rest of this chapter.

The Good News: It Isn't All Bad

In determining a person's heart disease risk, some experts say it's not total cholesterol but levels of LDL and HDL that matter most. LDL and HDL are lipoproteins, combinations of fat and protein made by the body. Lipoproteins are responsible for delivering cholesterol and other fats, which don't dissolve in the blood, to cells.

LDL, or low-density lipoprotein, carries most of the cholesterol in the blood. When there's too much LDL, it can combine with other substances to form a plaque, a hard, thick deposit that sticks to artery walls. If a blood clot develops in the vicinity of a plaque, the reduced blood flow can lead to a heart attack (or, if the affected artery feeds the brain, a stroke). This is why LDL is often described as the bad cholesterol.

HDL, or high-density lipoprotein, is known as the good cholesterol. It carries about one-third to one-fourth of the cholesterol in the blood, transporting it from different organs to the liver for disposal from the body. HDL may also pick up cholesterol deposited in your arteries and carry it to the liver.

Since research indicates that a high level of HDL can reduce your risk of heart attack, a healthy cholesterol profile would pair high HDL with low LDL. A routine cholesterol test would most likely measure HDL and LDL, as well as total cholesterol, for the most complete picture of your heart health.

++

When "Normal" Isn't Normal

In the past, standards for many health-related measures were determined by the average for the general population. Recently, though, some researchers have proposed that certain "normal" or "borderline" test results for cholesterol (as well as for triglycerides and blood pressure) may actually be unhealthy—and could be early warning signs for heart disease.

The American Heart Association recommends total cholesterol of less than 200 mg/dL (milligrams per deciliter), LDL of less than 130 mg/dL (the upper end of the near-optimal range), and HDL of 40 mg/dL or more. While experts don't agree on which numbers are best, it does look as though lower total cholesterol is better. In a study of 6,500 Chinese with an average total cholesterol of 127 mg/dL (compared with our 203 mg/dL), the death rate from heart disease was almost 17 times less for men and 6 times less for women. The Chinese ate half as much fat and one-tenth as much meat as Americans.

Most experts believe that your total cholesterol isn't the most important number, since a high level of HDL—the good kind—can drive up your cholesterol reading. The Framingham Cardiovascular Institute in Massachusetts urges its patients to focus on their levels of LDL—the bad kind—and their ratios of total cholesterol to HDL, which may be the most accurate gauge of heart health. The Institute recommends aiming for LDL below 110 and a total cholesterol/HDL ratio of less than 4 to 1.

++

Why the Big Deal about Cholesterol?

Keeping tabs on your cholesterol profile is your best insurance against coronary heart disease, the leading cause of death among men and women in the United States. The landmark Framingham Heart Study determined that the higher someone's total cholesterol level, the greater that person's heart disease risk. On the other hand, reducing total cholesterol by just 1 percent can reduce heart disease risk by 1 to 2 percent.

In coronary heart disease, the arteries that service the heart become narrowed by those LDL-deposited plaques. Studies suggest that plaques are most likely to develop on the walls of arteries that have been severely damaged. This damage can result from many things—not just LDL but also stress hormones, high blood pressure, uncontrolled diabetes, smoking, and a sedentary lifestyle.

When an artery becomes blocked and bloodflow is impeded, the heart muscle is deprived of oxygen. This causes chest pain, or angina. Some people experience angina only when they're exerting themselves or when they're under stress, since both situations increase the heart's demand for blood.

When bloodflow to the heart is severely limited, it can set the stage for a heart attack. In the most common scenario, a plaque in an artery that feeds the heart ruptures and triggers a blood clot.

++

The New Science of Heart Disease

Experts once thought that atherosclerosis, the buildup of cholesterol-packed plaque in the arteries that service the heart, was a lot like rust in an old pipe. Therefore, they reasoned, controlling cholesterol could reduce heart attack risk the way a weekly dose of drain cleaner prevents clogged pipes.

Now they're realizing their theory may have been too simplistic. According to groundbreaking new research, the buildup of plaque often begins when the smooth cells lining artery walls are injured or irritated. The culprits include LDL cholesterol that has been oxidized (altered by renegade molecules called free radicals); homocysteine, a naturally occurring amino acid; and apo B, a protein that carries cholesterol into artery walls.

Many of these recently discovered risk factors can be checked using new tests. While they won't replace regular cholesterol testing, they will provide valuable information about the state of your heart health. If you have other risk factors for heart disease, you may want to discuss these tests with your doctor.

Homocysteine: Having some of this amino acid in your blood is normal and apparently harmless. But more than a dozen studies suggest that slightly elevated levels—above 9 micromoles per liter—may greatly raise your risk for a heart attack or stroke, even when your cholesterol levels are normal.

The Abbott homocysteine test costs about $80, depending on your insurance carrier. Test results are available within hours.

Apolipoprotein A-1 (apo A-1) and apolipoprotein B (apo B): These two substances speed through the bloodstream carrying chunks of cholesterol. Apo A-1 rounds up potentially heart-harming fats and delivers them to the liver, while apo B carries cholesterol to artery walls and leaves it behind.

The riskiest situation is having a low level of apo A-1 and a high level of apo B. One study of 1,000 people showed that this combination quadrupled the odds of a second heart attack. It may be bad news even for people who haven't had a heart attack.

Consult your doctor about the test for apo A-1 and apo B, which costs $100 to $120.

Lipoprotein (a): No one knows the purpose of lipoprotein (a), or LP(a), which is basically a cholesterol chunk wrapped in a protein coat. Several studies, including one at Oxford University in England, have established an association between a high LP(a) level and an elevated heart disease risk.

Ask your doctor about having your LP(a) level checked. Specialized laboratories will administer the test for about $75.

C-reactive protein (CRP): This substance is produced in the liver when arteries are inflamed. It's a kind of early-warning system, with high levels indicating whether plaque is likely to rupture. In the Harvard Physicians' Health Study, high levels of CRP predicted a first heart attack 6 to 8 years in advance and were associated with a threefold increase in risk.

Ask for the high-sensitivity CRP (hs-CRP) test, not a standard CRP test, which is used for diagnosing conditions such as arthritis and inflammatory bowel disease. The test costs $60 and is widely available.

+++

The Rules of the Numbers Game

Clearly, coronary heart disease is serious business. But in many cases, it can be prevented, just by keeping high cholesterol under control. Above all else, that means getting your cholesterol checked on a regular basis.

The test is done on a blood sample from your finger or arm. The resulting measurements are expressed as milligrams per deciliter (mg/dL) of blood. For a test of total cholesterol and HDL levels, you don't need to fast beforehand. For a complete lipid profile, which measures total cholesterol, HDL, LDL, and triglycerides (a type of blood fat), you must fast for 9 to 12 hours. That means no food and no beverages except water, black coffee, or tea.

The National Cholesterol Education Program, an initiative of the National Heart, Lung, and Blood Institute, advises everyone age 20 and over to get their cholesterol checked at least once every 5 years. For men over 45 and women over 55, more frequent testing may be in order, since cholesterol levels tend to rise with age. Once you receive your results, your doctor will likely recommend a retest if any of your numbers are cause for concern.

To interpret your cholesterol profile, the American Heart

Association (AHA) offers the following guidelines. (For triglyceride numbers, see "Triglycerides: The Other Blood Fat" on page 19.)

FOR TOTAL CHOLESTEROL

> *Desirable:* less than 200 mg/dL
>
> *Borderline:* 200 to 239 mg/dL
>
> *High:* 240 mg/dL or higher

If your total cholesterol is less than 200 mg/dL and you have no other risk factors, you're not very likely to develop heart disease. On the other hand, a reading in the borderline range is reason for caution. Even if you have no other risk factors, you should try to get your total cholesterol below 200 mg/dL.

If your total cholesterol falls in the high category, it's definitely a red flag. It means you're even more likely to develop heart disease than someone in the borderline category. You may be especially vulnerable if you have other risk factors. In this situation, your best bet is to consult your doctor about further testing and treatment options.

FOR LDL

> *Optimal:* less than 100 mg/dL
>
> *Near optimal/above optimal:* 100 to 129 mg/dL
>
> *Borderline high:* 130 to 159 mg/dL
>
> *High:* 160 to 189 mg/dL
>
> *Very high:* 190 mg/dL or higher

If your LDL reading is in the borderline-high or high categories, your doctor will evaluate your other risk factors to determine whether you need to lower your LDL level.

FOR HDL

Desirable: 40 mg/dL or higher

On average, men have HDL in the range of 40 to 50 mg/dL; women, in the range of 50 to 60 mg/dL. Your doctor can tell you whether you need to raise your HDL level.

++

Triglycerides: The Other Blood Fat

When your doctor sends you for a cholesterol test, he may order a lipid profile, which measures total cholesterol, LDL, HDL, and triglycerides. You may wonder how triglycerides fit into the overall cholesterol picture.

Most fat in foods, and in your body, takes the form of triglycerides. When you consume more calories than you need, the extras are converted to triglycerides and stored in fat cells. Then later, when your body requires energy, certain hormones trigger the release of triglycerides to meet the demand.

Some research has shown that people with above-normal triglyceride levels are at increased risk for heart disease. They're also likely to have high total cholesterol, high LDL, and low HDL—all risk factors for heart disease.

The American Heart Association offers these guidelines for assessing triglyceride levels.

Normal: less than 150 mg/dL

Borderline high: 150 to 199 mg/dL

High: 200 to 499 mg/dL

Very high: greater than 500 mg/dL

If your triglycerides exceed 150 mg/dL, your doctor may recommend avoiding foods high in cholesterol and saturated fat, exercising regularly, and quitting smoking. You may also need to monitor your carbohydrate intake, since too many carbs can raise triglycerides while reducing HDL.

If your triglycerides top the 200 mark, you can still benefit from lifestyle changes. But you may also need medications to reduce your triglycerides to a healthier level. Your doctor can help determine the best course of treatment.

++

CHOLESTEROL RATIO

Some doctors believe that the ratio of total cholesterol to HDL is more accurate than total cholesterol alone as a marker for heart disease. To determine your ratio, divide your total cholesterol reading by your HDL reading. According to the AHA, the healthiest ratio is 3.5:1, but anything under 5:1 is acceptable.

The Rest of the Risk Factors

Not surprisingly, high cholesterol and heart disease have many risk factors in common. Some are beyond your control, such as your age (both high cholesterol and heart attacks are more likely as you get older) and your family history (genes help determine how your body handles LDL cholesterol). But others, including the following, can be minimized simply by making the right lifestyle choices.

Diet: You can make a big difference in your cholesterol profile, and your heart disease risk, just by reducing your consumption of animal products such as meats and dairy products. They're loaded with cholesterol and saturated fat, which are no good for your heart. Also be wary of oils high in saturated fat—especially coconut oil, palm kernel oil, and palm oil, which are common in processed foods.

Once in your bloodstream, saturated fat prevents LDL from properly breaking down in the liver, which in turn drives your LDL level higher. Even low-cholesterol or cholesterol-free foods may be bad for you if they contain an abundance of saturated fat.

Physical inactivity: If you have high cholesterol and you've been sedentary, one of the best things you can do for your heart is get moving. Among its many benefits, regular exercise can lower your LDL level, raise your HDL level, and help you maintain a healthy weight. Physical activity can also control other risk factors for heart disease, including high blood pressure.

Smoking: If you smoke, you're more than twice as likely as a nonsmoker to have a heart attack. That's because cigarette smoke oxidizes LDL, making it more likely to form artery-clogging plaque. Motivate yourself to banish the butts with the knowledge that within 2 years of quitting, your risk of heart attack drops to the level of someone who never smoked at all.

Overweight: Too much body fat often means too much LDL cholesterol, but slimming down can reduce the risk of heart disease. Excess pounds not only strain your heart, they also affect your blood pressure and increase your odds of developing diabetes.

Stress: While the role of stress in high cholesterol and heart disease isn't clear, unhealthy responses to stress—such as overeating and smoking—are recognized risk factors.

High blood pressure and diabetes: Both of these conditions raise your risk of heart disease. If you have either one, you should be under professional care. Your doctor can monitor your health status and adjust your treatment as necessary.

++

His-and-Hers Heart Health

Although heart disease is equally deadly for men and for women, it expresses itself differently in the two sexes. The risk among men is greater, and they have heart attacks earlier. But the death rate among women who have first heart attacks is twice as high as among men of the same age.

Beginning at menopause, a woman's risk of heart disease slowly rises, until eventually, it's the same as for a man. Premature menopause (before age 38)—either natural or surgical—increases the risk of heart attack, as does taking birth control pills in combination with smoking.

++

Remember: You're in Control

If high cholesterol has a bright side, it's that the condition not only is manageable but can be reversible. You have a multitude of treatments at your disposal to help you do just that. Some are basic lifestyle strategies, like redesigning your diet and establishing a fitness routine. Others are sophisticated new drugs. Your doctor can help you decide which treatment, or combination of treatments, will work best for you.

Research has proven that reducing cholesterol levels can help prevent heart attacks and heart attack deaths. In a Scandinavian study involving a statin, a widely prescribed cholesterol-lowering drug, the participants experienced a 25 percent reduction in total cholesterol and a 35 percent reduction in LDL cholesterol. In turn, the death rate for the group dropped by 42 percent, the likelihood of nonfatal heart attacks by 37 percent, and the need for heart surgery (bypass or angioplasty) by 37 percent.

These impressive numbers underscore just how lifesaving cholesterol control can be. With the strategies described in the following chapters and the guidance of your doctor, you can achieve better cholesterol readings and enjoy a longer, healthier life.

TREATMENTS
YOUR HEART WILL LOVE

✦ ✦ ✦

No one questions that high cholesterol has some serious implications for heart health. Still, committing to a treatment plan can be a challenge. Perhaps that's because high cholesterol produces no outward symptoms. It doesn't make you feel sick or exhausted. And so it goes about its artery-clogging business without any outside intervention.

If you've been diagnosed with a cholesterol problem, you can't wait for warning signs of heart disease to prod you into action. Two research groups, the Framingham Heart Study and the National Heart, Lung, and Blood Institute, found that 50 percent men and 63 percent of women who died suddenly of coronary heart disease had no prior symptoms of illness.

Yes, reining in your cholesterol takes hard work and commitment. But it's worth the effort, especially if you can protect yourself from something as devastating—and potentially deadly—as a heart attack or stroke.

From the remedies presented here, and with guidance from your doctor, you can build a cholesterol treatment plan that you can live with. You may be surprised at how even minor lifestyle changes can produce major improvements in your cholesterol profile.

Start with the Basics

These days, doctors aren't quite as quick to prescribe cholesterol-lowering medication for people with low to moderate risk of heart disease. Instead, they'll instruct these patients to improve their eating habits, increase their physical activity, and shed any extra pounds they may be carrying. By themselves, this trio of strategies may be enough to whip an unhealthy cholesterol profile into shape.

Of the three, diet may have the greatest influence on cholesterol levels, for better or for worse. In this country, we tend to eat lots of foods with lots of dietary cholesterol and saturated fat, both of which drive blood cholesterol upward. Interestingly, though, it's saturated fat—not dietary cholesterol—that bears most of the responsibility for clogging arteries.

While not quite as influential as diet, both a sedentary lifestyle and overweight contribute to high cholesterol and coronary heart disease. So working out and slimming down may not only improve your cholesterol profile but also reduce your heart attack risk.

If these changes don't produce the results you want within about 6 months, your doctor may recommend using a cholesterol-lowering medication. You can try a conventional pharmaceutical or try an alternative remedy—or both. As the rest of this chapter shows, you have plenty of options available. (*Note:* If you're considered at high risk for heart disease, your doctor has probably put you on cholesterol-lowering medication already. In your situation, that's really your best bet. Adding lifestyle changes, as well as some of the remedies that follow, may give you even better results, and more quickly.)

++

HRT and a Woman's Heart

Today, doctors are being a little more judicious about prescribing hormone replacement therapy (HRT) to menopausal women. Their new perspective was prompted by a large study in which HRT was found to actually increase the risk of death among women who already have heart disease.

What's more, preliminary results from the first large-scale, controlled clinical trial to examine the relationship between HRT and heart disease have revealed that women on HRT are at slightly higher risk for heart-related problems, including heart attack and stroke. (Other studies suggest that HRT increases breast cancer risk, too.)

Since these findings are based on early experience, experts don't rule out the possibility that HRT has long-term benefits. And while they won't know for certain until other studies are completed in 2005, many believe that HRT is safe—and beneficial—if you have risk factors for heart disease but haven't yet developed the condition.

Your best bet is to discuss HRT with your doctor before menopause, so you'll have a plan in place. If you're already taking HRT, experts advise against discontinuing it based on the research findings to date. If you've been diagnosed with heart disease, on the other hand, you should consider other options for managing your menopausal discomforts.

++

Medications: The Mainstream
Treatment of Choice

While cholesterol-lowering medications abound, three categories are most popular: the bile acid resins, a form of niacin (a B vitamin), and the statins. All three lower LDL, which is important because high LDL has the most serious impact on heart disease risk. Niacin also lowers total cholesterol and triglycerides while raising HDL.

Bile acid resins: These medications "pick up" cholesterol-containing bile acids in the intestines and carry them out of the body. This reduces LDL levels by 10 to 20 percent—or by more than 40 percent when the resins are taken in combination with statins.

Two commonly prescribed resins are cholestyramine (Prevalite) and colestipol (Colestid). Although both drugs appear safe for long-term use, they can cause gas, bloating, constipation, and nausea. Experts recommend mixing the powder form with water or fruit juice; if you're taking the tablets, wash them down with lots of water to prevent gastrointestinal side effects. Also, if you're on any other medications, take them either 1 hour before or 4 to 6 hours after the resins, since the resins may affect their absorption.

Niacin: In high daily doses of 1,000 to 3,000 milligrams, niacin has been shown to dramatically improve the entire cholesterol profile. In studies, it has lowered LDL by 10 to 25 percent, raised HDL by 15 to 35 percent, and decreased triglycerides by 20 to 50 percent.

Niacin lowers LDL by partially blocking the release of fatty acids from fat tissue, and by limiting the liver's production of VLDL (very low density lipoprotein). Since VLDL is partially converted to LDL, reducing it generates a corresponding decline in LDL.

++

Should You Take Aspirin?

For more than a dozen years, doctors have recommended an aspirin a day to ward off a second heart attack. But a Harvard study has found that among people over age 40 with heart disease, only 47 percent of men and 36 percent of women actually use aspirin, despite its proven benefits. And as many as a million people may be forgoing aspirin in favor of acetaminophen and ibuprofen, which do not offer the same protection.

Aspirin helps prevent blood platelet clumping, which can lead to dangerous clots. It may also reduce blood vessel inflammation. To find out if you should use it, see your doctor. Generally, you may benefit if you meet one of the following criteria.

- You've already had a heart attack. Taking 80 milligrams a day, the equivalent of one low-dose aspirin, can reduce your risk of a second heart attack by 25 percent.

- You haven't had a heart attack, but you have other risk factors for heart disease. Your doctor can tell you whether they warrant using aspirin therapy.

- You don't have gastrointestinal problems. Long-term use of aspirin can lead to bleeding and gastric upset. You can avoid these side effects by taking an enteric-coated product.

Note: Aspirin is a nonsteroidal anti-inflammatory drug, or NSAID. If you take another NSAID—such as ibuprofen for arthritis—check with your doctor about the safety of adding a low-dose aspirin.

++

You can buy niacin over the counter, but the high doses necessary for cholesterol control are available only by prescription. They must be supervised by a physician to guard against possible serious liver side effects. Make sure you're taking nicotinic acid, since the form called nicotinamide or niacinamide has no effect on cholesterol.

Although at least one study has linked niacin with liver abnormalities, more recent research suggests that as long as it's given in the proper dose, such complications are relatively rare. Still, while you're on niacin, your doctor should monitor your liver enzymes.

The other troublesome side effect of niacin is the flushing that most people who take it initially experience. It should subside as your body adjusts. In addition, research indicates that flushing can be eliminated in 80 percent of cases by taking niacin with meals; avoiding alcohol, spicy foods, and hot liquids; and not skipping doses. Some niacin is designed to be taken at bedtime so any flushing occurs while you sleep.

In some people, niacin therapy triggers high blood sugar and gout. Your doctor may not prescribe niacin if you already have diabetes or high uric acid levels (which contribute to gout).

If your cholesterol level is exceptionally high, you and your doctor may want to consider combining niacin with a statin.

Statins: Some of the most widely prescribed cholesterol-lowering drugs, statins work by slowing the body's production of cholesterol and helping the liver to remove LDL that's already in the blood. Studies have linked statins with 20 to 60 percent reductions in LDL, along with slight increases in HDL and declines in triglycerides. Six statin drugs are currently available: lovastatin (Mevacor), simvastatin (Zocor), pravastatin (Pravachol), fluvastatin (Lescol), atorvastatin (Lipitor), and cerivastatin (Baycol).

Once you've been taking this medication for 6 to 8 weeks,

your doctor will probably send you for a cholesterol test, then average those results with a second test to see how the statin is working. Because your body produces more cholesterol at night, plan to take your medication in the early evening or at bedtime.

The potential side effects of statins include mild discomforts such as gas, upset stomach, constipation, and abdominal cramps. These should disappear as your body adjusts to treatment. Rarely, liver abnormalities and muscle problems can also develop.

Supplements: Nutritional Heart Helpers

Aside from niacin, with its powerful cholesterol-reducing action, several other nutrients can support your anti-cholesterol campaign. Some of these vitamins and minerals are antioxidants; they don't actually lower cholesterol, but they prevent LDL from oxidizing, so it doesn't harden and clog arteries. Among the supplements you may want to consider are vitamin C, vitamin E, and chromium. Be sure to ask your doctor about them before beginning supplementation.

Vitamin C: Dozens of studies have linked high blood levels of vitamin C with lower total cholesterol and triglycerides, as well as higher HDL. In one study, people with low blood levels of vitamin C who took 1,000 milligrams of the nutrient a day experienced an average 7 percent increase in HDL over the course of 8 months.

Prevention magazine recommends taking 100 to 500 milligrams of vitamin C daily, in addition to the amount in your multivitamin/mineral supplement. Be aware that doses above 2,000 milligrams a day can cause diarrhea in some people.

Vitamin E: For a person with heart disease, taking vitamin E supplements may reduce the risk of death by 40 to 60 percent. As an antioxidant, vitamin E prevents LDL from oxidizing.

Many doctors recommend taking 400 international units of vitamin E a day. Because it acts as a blood thinner, consult your doctor before beginning supplementation if you're already using a blood-thinning medication such as aspirin or warfarin (Coumadin).

Chromium: Though it's not an antioxidant, the mineral chromium may help control cholesterol. Experts theorize that it improves the efficiency of insulin, the hormone that helps the body metabolize blood sugar. Many studies show that when insulin levels are normal, so are cholesterol levels.

If you're interested in trying chromium, check with your doctor. Dosages above 1,000 micrograms require medical supervision.

+++

Know the Signs of a Heart Attack

Too often, people ignore the initial symptoms of a heart attack. And that's unfortunate, because the sooner they would seek medical attention, the less damage the heart muscle would suffer, and the greater their chances of recovery would be.

If you experience any of the following, chew a full-strength (325-milligram) aspirin—it may improve your survival rate in the event that you are having a heart attack—and call 911 or your area's emergency medical number immediately, advises Robert S. Rosenson, M.D., director of the preventive cardiology center at Northwestern University Medical School in Chicago.

For men: The classic symptom is uncomfortable pressure, fullness, squeezing, or pain in the center of the chest that lasts more than a few minutes or that quickly fades in and out. The pain may spread to the shoulders, neck, or arms, and it may be

accompanied by light-headedness, sweating, nausea, or shortness of breath.

For women: The pain tends to be lighter than in men, and it
may affect the chest, stomach, or abdomen. Other symptoms
include nausea or dizziness, shortness of breath, heart palpitations, fatigue, and weakness.

At the hospital, if you're examined and told your heart is fine,
insist on a thorough evaluation, including an electrocardiogram.
It's not all that uncommon for patients who have heart disease
to be sent home from the ER with a clean bill of health.

+++

Herbs: Mother Nature's Cholesterol Medicines

Several herbal remedies have longstanding reputations as
gentle, effective treatments for high cholesterol. And they
have the scientific research to support their cholesterol-
lowering capabilities. Consider adding one—or more—of
the following to your anti-cholesterol arsenal.

Flaxseed: Flaxseed and flaxseed oil contain omega-3 fatty
acids, which are thought to protect the heart and artery walls
from the damage caused by high cholesterol. Experts suggest
taking 1½ tablespoons of ground flaxseed or 1 teaspoon of
flaxseed oil a day for as long as necessary.

If you use ground flaxseed, be sure to take it with at least 8
ounces of water. Don't take it at all if you have a bowel obstruction.

++

The Red Yeast Rice Debate

Perhaps one of the most controversial cholesterol treatments is red yeast rice, which was formerly sold under the brand name Cholestin. The product contained substances that were similar to prescription statin drugs, and trials showed that it could dramatically lower cholesterol.

Now, Cholestin has been taken off the market following the FDA's decision that it infringed on patents for lovastatin, a prescription drug sold as Mevacor. Generic red yeast rice is still available, but it should be used very cautiously. Many of the generic products aren't as well-studied as Cholestin, and they tend to contain lower levels of the cholesterol-lowering compounds, according to Andrew Weil, M.D., director of the program in integrative medicine at the University of Arizona in Tucson. Also, if you're taking any medication, be sure to talk to your doctor before trying red yeast rice. The herb isn't appropriate for people under age 20, women who are pregnant or nursing, or people with a history of liver disease.

++

Garlic: Since HDL directs excess cholesterol out of your body, you want to keep your HDL level high. Garlic can help you do just that. Consumed regularly, garlic can also lower total cholesterol, as numerous studies have shown.

Experts recommend eating a clove or more a day or taking two to four 300- to 400-milligram capsules a day. Look for a product labeled as providing 4,000 micrograms of allicin potential per capsule. (Allicin is the principal active constituent in garlic.)

Because garlic thins the blood and may increase bleeding, you don't want to take supplements if you're already on blood-thinning drugs or if you're scheduled for surgery. Likewise, you should avoid garlic if you're on medication to lower your blood sugar.

Green tea and black tea: Natural compounds called flavonoids, found in tea as well as in many fruits and vegetables, have a protective effect on the heart. The flavonoids in four to five cups of green or black tea a day can help keep cholesterol from sticking to your arteries. To maximize the flavonoid content of your tea, use tea bags instead of loose leaves and steep for 5 minutes.

If you don't like green tea, you can buy green leaf extract in capsules at health food stores. Take 100 milligrams three times daily. Avoid using medicinal doses of black tea for an extended period of time, as it may stimulate the nervous system.

Guggul: Native to India, the guggul tree yields a gummy resin that lowers LDL and raises HDL. The powdered extract is available in capsule form, and the standard recommended dosage is three 1,000-milligram capsules containing 2.5 percent guggulsterones a day, with meals.

Once your cholesterol profile improves, you still need to continue taking guggul (which may be labeled as gugulipid) unless you make serious lifestyle changes. In rare cases, the herb may trigger diarrhea, restlessness, or hiccups.

Hawthorn: Experts believe hawthorn to be the best herb overall for heart health. Some research suggests that it lowers cholesterol, too.

Look for a product made with hawthorn extract that's standardized to contain 1.8 percent of a compound called vitexin. Take 100 milligrams three times a day.

Anyone with a heart condition should not take hawthorn regularly for more than a few weeks without medical supervision. Your doctor may need to adjust your dosage of other medications. Likewise, if you have low blood pressure caused by heart valve problems, do not use hawthorn without medical supervision.

++

A Toast to Good Health

The next time you order wine with your dinner, think red. According to laboratory studies, compounds in red wine slow the oxidation of both HDL and LDL cholesterol. This preventive effect may be doubly good: Oxidation not only lowers your HDL cholesterol, it also seems to encourage the formation of plaque in your arteries.

The key is to keep your alcohol consumption moderate. For women, that means no more than one 5-ounce glass of wine a day; for men, no more than two 5-ounce glasses a day. Of course, if you don't already drink, don't start just to improve your cholesterol profile.

++

Foods: Edible Heart Protection

You know what *not* to eat when you're trying to rein in your cholesterol. But you may not realize that certain foods can help improve your cholesterol profile. Some of these good guys may surprise you.

Beans: The soluble fiber in beans can help lower cholesterol by enhancing the intestines' ability to excrete it. And because beans are a protein, they're an excellent substitute for other protein sources that are higher in fat and cholesterol, such as meats.

Extra-virgin olive oil: In one study, extra-virgin (unrefined) olive oil did a better job than refined olive oil in stopping LDL from oxidizing. The theory is that the high levels of antioxidants in the oil may slow the formation of arterial plaques.

Fish: Fish is much lower in saturated fat and cholesterol than red meat or poultry, so substituting it for those foods may help keep LDL from rising to an unhealthy level. Fatty fish like salmon, mackerel, and herring contain omega-3 fatty acids, which studies have shown may help protect against heart disease. Try for a minimum of two 6-ounce servings of fish a week, as recommended by the American Heart Association.

If you can't work fish into your diet, you may want to try fish oil supplements that provide about 1 gram of omega-3 fatty acids per day.

Nuts: Because nuts are rich in "good fats," vitamin E, and phytochemicals, eating a handful several times a week may help reduce heart disease risk. Just don't overindulge, or you'll gain weight.

++

Eat, Drink . . . but Be Wary

We're frequently warned to watch out for interactions between various medications we may be taking. But even healthful foods like broccoli can cause similar problems.

In some cases, a food can make a drug either less effective or more powerful. In other cases, mixing a food and a drug can lead to unwanted side effects. For example, high-potassium foods such as broccoli can interact with the potassium-sparing diuretics used to treat high blood pressure, causing the mineral to build up in the body. Too much potassium can trigger an irregular heartbeat and palpitations.

The following list highlights drugs prescribed for heart-related problems and the foods that may interact with them.

- Digoxin (Lanoxin), prescribed for congestive heart failure and atrial fibrillation, may interact with bran fiber that decreases absorption of the drug. Take digoxin apart from meals.

- Warfarin (Coumadin), a blood thinner used for heart attack, atrial fibrillation, venous thrombosis, pulmonary embolism, and stroke, may interact with foods high in vitamin K, such as leafy greens and broccoli. Large amounts of the vitamin decrease the drug's effect, while too small amounts increase its effect. Aim for a consistent intake of vitamin K.

- Calcium channel blockers such as amlodipine (Norvasc), diltiazem (Cardizem), and nifedipine (Procardia or Adalat), prescribed for high blood pressure and congestive heart failure, may interact with grapefruit juice in a way that reduces the drugs' absorption. Avoid grapefruit juice for at least 2 hours before and 2 hours after taking any of these medications.

- Statin drugs such as simvastatin (Zocor), pravastatin (Pravachol), and atorvastatin (Lipitor), used for high cholesterol, may also interact with grapefruit juice. If you're taking any of these drugs, you should stay away from alcohol, since excess consumption may increase the risk of liver damage.

++

Orange juice: In one study, people who drank three glasses of OJ a day saw their heart-helping HDL increase by

21 percent. While researchers aren't completely sure why orange juice had this effect, they suspect a flavonoid called hesperidin may play a role.

Peanut butter: Everybody's favorite spread is rich in mono-unsaturated fat, which has been shown to lower levels of LDL and triglycerides while preserving levels of HDL. If you increase your consumption of peanut products, be sure to pay attention to serving sizes and eat them in place of foods with similar calorie counts. (For example, 2 tablespoons of peanut butter or ¼ cup of peanuts has the same number of calories as 32 mini-pretzels or 18 baked potato chips.) Otherwise, you may put on pounds, which will negate any benefits to your heart.

Soy: Soy may lower both total cholesterol and LDL levels without reducing HDL levels, although scientists have yet to figure out how it works. One theory is that certain compounds in soy, called phytoestrogens, help transport LDL from the bloodstream to the liver, where it's broken down and excreted. Phytoestrogens may also keep LDL from oxidizing, so it's less likely to clog your arteries.

According to the Food and Drug Administration, eating about 25 grams of soy protein a day can help reduce cholesterol, compared with eating animal protein. You can get soy protein from products such as soy milk, tofu, and soy nuts.

Make Your Treatment Plan Stick

While all of the treatments mentioned in this chapter can help improve your cholesterol profile, none of them is a quick fix. Managing your cholesterol takes time and commitment, from you and your doctor.

Your doctor's mission is to provide you with the information you need and to monitor your health along the way. Your mission is to implement whatever strategies might benefit you in your unique situation: Eat a more healthful diet, establish an exercise program, stop smoking or lose weight if necessary, faithfully take any medications that you're prescribed, and try some of the remedies suggested here (in consultation your doctor, of course). All of these measures have been tested, and they're scientifically proven to work.

To help you stay with your individual program, set short-term goals you feel you can achieve, then enlist support by discussing your goals with your doctor and the people closest to you. If you find you're having trouble attaining a particular goal, analyze the reasons and come up with an alternate plan that will help you succeed.

In the following chapters, you'll read about the experiences of people who confronted their own struggles with high cholesterol and overcame them. Let their stories inspire you to take action.

EAT WELL TO WIN

✦ ✦ ✦

HER MEALS GET
HER UNDIVIDED ATTENTION

In the years in which she has been working to rein in her own cholesterol, Grace Penny has made an interesting observation. "Most people don't allow themselves to truly enjoy eating," she says. "They gulp down their food and then go about their business, as though ignoring the fact that they've eaten might prevent them from gaining weight."

Grace knows what she's talking about. The 65-year-old retired teacher from Lutz, Florida, used to disconnect from her diet. Then a revolutionary weight-loss program taught her how to pay attention to what she put her mouth. She not only shed pounds, she also cut her cholesterol.

In 1996, Grace learned that she had type 2 (non-insulin-dependent) diabetes as well as high cholesterol. Her LDL was a dangerously high 220; her HDL, a too-low 25; and her total cholesterol, a high 254. Her doctor prescribed medication for both conditions, but Grace disliked being dependent on prescription drugs.

Two years later, Grace made a decision that would change the course of her health—and her life. "I had just gotten back from a 2-mile walk, and I felt so disgusted because I was out of breath," she recalls. "That's when I made up my mind to enroll in the Rice Diet Program."

Based at Duke University in Durham, North Carolina, the Rice Diet Program aims to improve its clients' health with a low-salt, low-fat diet as well as mind-body training techniques. Grace found the residential treatment facility through an Internet search. Initially, she spent a month there, following a very restricted eating plan and attending classes on everything from nutrition to water aerobics to meditation.

Of all that she learned in the program, Grace was most fascinated by the exercises in mindful eating. "When you eat mindfully, you take time to savor every bite of food," she explains. "You taste it and smell it. You look at it and think about the source, the preparation, the presentation, the color. You also pay attention to the surroundings—the dishes, the table, the room, the people you're eating with."

One exercise required Grace to spend a full 10 to 15 minutes dining on three raisins. In another exercise—a "mindful lunch" organized by the program instructors—Grace had 45 minutes to eat a cup of steamed spinach, a cup of steamed carrots, and a large apple. "The idea is to listen to our bodies and identify our individual satiation points," Grace explains. "After that lunch, I felt full. And I was only mildly hungry by dinnertime."

Of course, Grace doesn't always eat that slowly. But she does make an effort to eat mindfully at every meal. "As long as I stay tuned in to my body, I know when I'm full, and I don't overeat," she says. "I think that's been a major factor in helping me to slim down and to lower my cholesterol."

Indeed, within 1 week of enrolling in the Rice Diet Program, Grace was able to wean herself from Lipitor and Glucotrol, medications she had been taking for cholesterol and diabetes, respectively. Within 7 months, she dropped from 205 to 155 pounds (she's 5 feet ¾ inch tall). By 2000, her total cholesterol had reached a healthy level.

Every 6 months, Grace goes back to Duke University for 1- to 2-week follow-up sessions. Her latest blood test puts her total cholesterol at 187, her LDL at 100, and her HDL at 43—all dramatic improvements. Her triglycerides remain high at 220, but Grace is thrilled that they've dropped from 305 without medication. Since March 1998, when she enrolled in the Rice Diet Program, she's also lost more weight; at 140, she's getting ever closer to her goal of 115 to 120.

WINNING ACTION

Spend time savoring every spoonful. When you take a bite of food, your brain doesn't get the message for a full 20 minutes. You could conceivably eat an entire meal, and then some, before your brain lets you know you're stuffed. That sets the stage for overeating, which can contribute to weight gain as well as cholesterol trouble. At meals, chew your food slowly, all the while focusing on the taste, the smell, the color—the very act of eating. You'll notice that you feel full on much less, and you'll stay satisfied longer.

++

HE HAS A NEW CREDO: "BEFORE YOU EAT IT, KNOW WHAT IT IS"

Jim McDonnell's kids used to love when he grocery shopped. "All the junk they wanted to eat, I would buy for them," says Jim, 69, a retired insurance sales manager from Salisbury Township, Pennsylvania. "Now, I don't put anything in the basket without reading the label. I have learned to eat smart."

In 1997, Jim's cholesterol hovered around 300. But he was not worried about it, until he started experiencing muscle weakness in his legs caused by an arterial blockage. In early 2000, he had his right carotid artery operated on to clean out plaque buildup. "It was even more serious than the testing indicated," he says.

After the surgery, his doctor recommended that he participate in a cholesterol reduction study taking place at Lehigh Valley Hospital. It's called LOVAR (Lowering of Vascular Atherosclerotic Risk) and combines nutrition and exercise classes with medication. Jim takes Pravachol, Plavix (an aspirin substitute), a multivitamin, and supplements of vitamins C and E, folic acid, calcium, magnesium, and zinc.

Following the advice of a physical therapist, he has built up to 30 minutes a day on the treadmill, at between 2.6 and 2.8 miles per hour and at an incline setting of 3. When he started the treadmill a year ago, he could go only 2 minutes on it before having to rest.

After 4 months of nutrition classes, he cut way back on red meat. He replaced high-fat ice cream with nonfat frozen yogurt, increased his vegetable and fruit intake to nine servings a day, and learned to check out the fat content and ingredients of products before buying them. "Before, I never gave that one iota of thought," he says. "I was a lazy eater. Anything I could put in my mouth, I put in."

At his most recent screening, his cholesterol was 230—still too high, he says. "I want to get to 200." On the plus side, he has lost 10 pounds. He's 5 feet 11, and he did weigh 190. Now he's only 5 pounds from his goal of 175.

"I used to think nothing about a couple of doughnuts for breakfast," Jim says. "I didn't really know what was in them, nutrition-wise. Now I know." These days, breakfast is a bowl of bran cereal or oatmeal with a soy–cow's milk blend.

Lunch, at one time a cheeseburger or a sandwich "with any kind of meat," is now a tuna sandwich with light mayonnaise. Steak for dinner has been replaced with lean meat and vegetables flavored with a cholesterol-lowering margarine.

"I used to be a big snacker," he adds. "I don't snack anymore."

Jim says that he feels great. He is happy to be able to enjoy trips to New York City and Europe with his wife, Bunny.

"Hardly a week goes by that I don't hear of a friend having a health problem," he says. "Maybe it is because of their lifestyle. They are doing the very thing I was doing: too much of what's not good for you."

WINNING ACTION

Understand what you're putting in your mouth. Too many tasty and easy-to-eat foods—packaged cookies, doughnuts, potato chips, fast-food cheeseburgers—are loaded with fat. And "low-cholesterol" or "no-cholesterol" claims don't mean that the foods can't be loaded with hydrogenated oils, which may be no better for you than animal fats. Your first step toward eating better is understanding how food ingredients affect your cholesterol. The second step is making sure the undesirable ingredients are not hidden in the snacks you love. As always, diligent label reading is essential. When you really understand that something is not good for you, the temptation to eat it fades.

++

FOR THE RECORD, SHE'S DOWN 100 POINTS

Helen Hurly could tell you exactly what she ate for breakfast yesterday, whether she lunched on a sandwich or a salad last

Tuesday, and if she snacked on a cookie anytime in the past month. While she may have a razor-sharp memory, she prefers to track every morsel in her food diary.

By keeping the diary, Helen—a 59-year-old sales analyst from Laurel, Maryland—hopes to better understand how various dietary strategies influence her cholesterol level. Her ultimate goal is to wean herself from Zocor, which she has been taking since 1998.

Helen never had a problem with her cholesterol until she turned 50. Then it never stopped climbing—from 212 to 240 and, eventually, 287. She had good reason to be concerned. "Both my parents died from strokes," she says. "And they weren't much older than I am now."

Once Helen's cholesterol reached 287, her doctor put her on Zocor. Within 3 months, her cholesterol plummeted almost 100 points, to 197. Helen was happy with the results, but she had no intention of staying on Zocor for the rest of her life. "I just didn't like the idea of taking a pill every day," she explains.

Because she had an established fitness routine—she still takes step aerobics four times a week—Helen decided to focus on her diet. She began by paying more attention to food labels. Then she came up with the idea of a food diary as a means of tracking her eating habits. "I bought a diary in which I could make notes every hour of every day," she says. "It turned out to be really eye-opening. Some days, I thought I was being really good. Then I'd look in my diary and see that I had eaten a cookie and two pieces of fudge. A sweet here, a strip of bacon there . . . it could really add up."

Helen's diary has proven especially valuable in assessing the effectiveness of various cholesterol-lowering diets she has tried. "I get my cholesterol checked every 3 months," she says. "Based on the results, I can look back through my diary to see what I did differently and whether it made my cholesterol profile better or worse. If a change seems to produce an improvement, I keep it up."

Sometimes this process yields surprising results. Once, for example, Helen tried strictly curtailing her fat intake. "I looked at my diary, as did my doctor," she says. "Both of us noticed that when I was following a very low fat diet, my numbers went up."

Helen remains careful about her fat intake, but she no longer aims for a totally fat-free diet. By using her food diary to continuously tweak her eating habits, she has lowered her total cholesterol to 187, with an LDL of about 98 and an HDL of about 60.

While many people would happily settle for this cholesterol profile, Helen believes she can do even better. That's why she's still keeping her food diary, still adjusting her diet until she finds what's best for her. "Everyone's biochemical makeup is unique," she says. "If you have high cholesterol, you've got to make choices and see how they affect you. I'm still doing that myself. I'm still taking Zocor, too—but hopefully, that will change soon."

WINNING ACTION

Take note of your meals and snacks. Many weight-loss experts recommend keeping a food diary in order to identify and adjust unhealthy eating patterns. This strategy can work just as well in a cholesterol management plan. You don't need an actual diary; an ordinary spiral-bound notebook will do. Keep it with you at all times. As soon as you eat something—even "just a snack"—write down what it is, when and where you're eating, and even how you're feeling. This way, you can develop a clearer picture of your diet and identify changes that may help bring your cholesterol under control.

+++

HE SEES HIS FUTURE
IN FOOD LABELS

Before Barrie Kissack puts any food item in his grocery cart, he scrutinizes the label, paying particular attention to fat and fiber content. If the item is not low-fat or high-fiber, it goes back on the shelf.

Reading all those labels takes time. But for Barrie, a 63-year-old educational consultant from Devon, England, it's worth the extra effort. It's helping him keep his cholesterol at a healthy level—and reduce his chances of another heart attack.

Barrie had his first heart attack in 1994. Back then, his total cholesterol measured 7.4 mmol/L, the British equivalent of about 287 mg/dL. He was also a bit heavier than he should have been, carrying 178 pounds on his 5-foot-8 frame.

To spare his heart further damage, Barrie knew that those numbers had to change. He consulted a nutritionist for guidance in developing a more heart-healthy diet. The nutritionist's advice was simple: If Barrie wanted to stop eating the wrong foods, he'd better stop bringing them home from the supermarket. "That made me start paying attention to food labels, which I had never done before," he says. "It certainly didn't require any willpower."

While Barrie scans all the nutrition information on the label, the fat and fiber contents tend to be the deciding factors in whether or not he buys a particular item. With fat, in particular, he never goes by large-print promises such as "reduced-fat" or "low-fat." He always checks the numbers for himself. "I think the most misleading phrase is '95% fat-free,'" he says. "In other words, that food is 5 percent fat. That's still too much for me."

When shopping for cereals, Barrie tries to stick with the highest-fiber brands. Neither muesli nor shredded wheat makes the cut, but oat and bran flakes usually do. In the dairy case, he chooses fat-free milk over low-fat, and skips butter in favor of a cholesterol-lowering spread such as Benecol.

Reading labels has had just the effect Barrie's nutritionist predicted: Now that Barrie is no longer bringing unhealthy foods into his home, he's eating more nutritiously than ever. Red meat is a rarity in the Kissack home, and if chicken is on the menu, Barrie's wife removes the skin before serving it. They prefer light lunches of soups and salads, and dinners with plenty of fruits and vegetables. Their favorite dessert, sponge pudding, has become a special treat instead of standard fare.

"Before, we hardly paid attention to what we were putting on our plates," Barrie says. "Now we think about what we're eating."

As he has become more conscientious about his food choices, Barrie has seen a positive impact on his cholesterol profile. His total cholesterol dropped to 6.4 mmol/L, or about 247 mg/dL, within 5 months of his heart attack. In Britain, that used to be considered a healthy level. Barrie also lost 34 pounds, which he has kept off.

By 2000, the British government had released updated cholesterol guidelines, setting 5 mmol/L—about 200 mg/dL—as the new desirable level. Barrie was able to achieve that goal with help from prescription statin drugs and continued vigilance about his food purchases and eating habits.

Barrie acknowledges that he spends extra time on grocery shopping, but he's perfectly content with his restyled diet. "In fact, I don't consider it a 'diet' in the conventional sense," he says. "I view it as a change for life."

WINNING ACTION

Peruse the label before purchasing. The "Nutrition Facts" labels that appear on almost all packaged foods contain a wealth of information, not just fat and fiber content. You can use these numbers to determine whether a particular item has a place in your cholesterol-lowering eating plan.

Just keep in mind that the "% Daily Value" figures for fat and calories are based on a 2,000-calorie-a-day diet. If you're consuming fewer calories than that, the "% Daily Value" figures increase proportionately.

++

HE WROTE HIMSELF A NEW MENU

By 1998, Ken Bombria had lived with high cholesterol for more than a decade. He kept promising his doctor that he'd improve his diet and get exercise, but the changes never stuck. Finally, his doctor put him on Zocor.

Within 3 weeks, his total cholesterol level had fallen to 220, but the damage was already done, and he soon had a heart attack. And that, says Ken, 58, "is what drives you to make changes."

While recovering, he discovered Dr. Dean Ornish's Program for Reversing Heart Disease and decided that it was the plan for him. He dropped red meat and egg yolks, switched to nonfat dairy products, and limited his fat intake to 10 percent of total calories within a plant-based eating plan.

At the suggestion of his cardiologist, Ken also eats 6-ounce portions of fish two or three times a week. "He believes that the omega-3 fatty acids in fish are vital to reducing cardiac disease," says Ken.

Ken, who lives in West Warren, Massachusetts, now realizes why his previous dieting efforts always failed. Before, he would limit his full-fat meals to three times a week and try to avoid fat the rest of the week. "If you're eating steak and eggs three times a week and no fat the rest of the time, the taste difference is huge," he says, especially since most nonfat recipes aren't that appetizing. This taste difference, says Ken, makes the fatty meals more enticing and the dieter more likely to splurge.

That's not the case anymore. "You learn how to add spices

and herbs to boost the flavor of the meal," says Ken, mentioning that he often uses three times the amount of spice listed in a recipe. "Once you become accustomed to the taste of these new dishes, it becomes your normal way of eating, and the foods taste really good."

Ken points out that since he, like most people, had only 8 to 10 meals that he rotated through, all he had to do was replace those core dishes to rework his entire diet. "When you change what you eat and how you stock your cupboard, you don't slide back into eating the fatty foods," he says.

For the rest of the Ornish program, Ken engages in 30 minutes of aerobic exercise and 30 minutes of resistance work on machines three times a week. He also practices a program of meditation daily. Two years after the heart attack that rearranged his life, Ken, at 5-feet-8, went from 215 pounds to 173, his total cholesterol fell to 132, and his LDL level dropped to an astonishingly low 68.

Ken still takes Zocor, but he knows there's no chance he'll return to his old, fat-eating ways. "If I drink milk that isn't fat-free, it tastes waxy in my mouth," he says. "Once you cleanse your palate, the fat doesn't even taste good. You really don't enjoy it."

WINNING ACTION

Rework your menu from top to bottom. You can try to limit yourself to just a couple of cookies or a steak once a week, but if the food is in the house, it will always be a temptation. Avoid the problem by developing a week's worth of meals that satisfy your cholesterol-lowering needs as well as your tastebuds, and keep other foods out of the house. As your palate adjusts to the new way of eating, you'll learn how to cook tasty and filling meals with ingredients that will keep your heart running strong.

++

HE'S WATCHING HIS FAT INTAKE
GRAM FOR GRAM

Randy Stoltzfus has spent a lifetime around food. As the owner and operator of three diners, he was accustomed to eating fatty fare, such as eggs, steak, and hamburgers. But these days, he lives by Randy's Rule: He doesn't eat anything with more than 1 gram of fat per serving. "I just made up my mind that's what I was going to do," says the 82-year-old Coopersburg, Pennsylvania, resident, whose cholesterol once hovered near 300.

It's a stringent rule for someone who had never given a moment's thought to the health impact of his dietary habits. "The food in diners tends to be high in fat and cholesterol, but I just ate anything I wanted," he says. "I didn't take any precautions."

All that began to change in the winter of 1987, when Randy experienced a squeezing sensation in his chest. "I was pushing snow off my back porch, " he recalls. "I wasn't even lifting it, just pushing it. I thought the tightness was not normal, so I went to see my doctor."

Within days, Randy underwent bypass surgery. At the time, his cholesterol was 289, and he weighed 192 pounds, more than enough for his 5-foot-7 frame. His doctor put him on the drug Zocor. In addition, he started taking Guggul Plus, an herbal supplement that contains guggulsterone, believed to help lower cholesterol. Two years after surgery, his cholesterol level had fallen to 235.

Determined to get it even lower, Randy made up his mind to avoid all foods with more than 1 gram of fat in a serving, regardless of serving size. "When I read and read some more, I decided to cut out the fat and see if it works," he says. "Well, it worked real well for me."

It took a few weeks to adjust to his new rule. "My daughter used to hate going to the store with me because I'd stop and read the cans, and she'd say it was a waste of time," Randy recalls. "But there's a lot of good stuff out there."

His vigilance paid off. Three years after his surgery, Randy's cholesterol fell to a low of 146. Another year later, his weight bottomed out at 140 pounds, where it's been ever since.

These days, Randy still works around food. He has a job at a sub shop, where he helps prepare subs but never eats them. He also passes on the potato nuggets and chips that accompany the subs, preferring instead to eat nothing at all or occasionally a veggie burger on a roll with low-fat cheese. "The roll has only half a gram of fat," he adds.

Randy shrugs off the difficulty involved in abiding by his rule. "You've got to make the move mentally," he says. "You just have to get it through your head that this is what you want to do."

WINNING ACTION

Impose a limit on how much fat you're going to eat, then stick with it. Fat, especially the saturated kind, is a primary culprit behind high cholesterol. Limiting yourself to a low fat intake, such as 1 gram per serving, makes it hard to get too much fat in your diet without overeating. Take the time to read labels on processed foods—you'll find more than you imagined to choose from. And learn which poultry, fish, and shellfish are lowest in fat. A 3-ounce serving of steamed shrimp, for instance, has only 0.9 gram. By setting a limit for yourself and learning which foods to avoid, you'll eat well and still lower your total cholesterol level.

++

HIS WIFE CUT THE FAT,
AND HE CUT HIS CHOLESTEROL

Neil Denbo, 71, had been fighting high cholesterol for more than a decade, with mixed results. It started back in 1990, when his doctor told him to change to a low-fat diet in response to a total cholesterol reading of 264.

"I cut back on fat calories, somewhat halfheartedly," Neil admits, yet he brought his total cholesterol down to 229 by the end of the year. Unfortunately, by 1991, the reading had climbed back to 252. "My level has bounced around since then," he says. "But there was no panic because I had a decent total cholesterol-to-HDL ratio, between 3.1 and 4.2."

Neil's doctor eventually put him on Zocor, but the medication didn't do much to alter his readings. In February 1998, for example, his total cholesterol was still 242.

The solution to Neil's changing cholesterol levels finally came in 1999, from a source he wouldn't have expected. "My wife, Arline, retired," he says, "and she has a different philosophy of running the kitchen. She started to tighten up on things."

Neil says that while he cooked with a lot of meat, "Arline wrings the fat out of everything. She's very interested in nutrition and how food reacts with your system." She used cooking sprays instead of butter or oil, eliminated egg yolks, and added a lot more grains, fruits, and vegetables. Most important, though, she took out a lot of the meat.

"We had beef stew the other night," says Neil, who lives in Gurnee, Illinois. "The recipe she was using called for 2 pounds of beef, but she used lean beef, put in half the amount, and added at least as many vegetables to make up for it.

"The way to trim back on the fat," he continues, "is not to put it in in the first place. Any meat that we use now, the ratio of vegetables to meat is three to one."

The Denbos also began walking together for an hour a day at 3½ miles per hour. By March 2000—with Neil taking Zocor and adding a margarine substitute called Benecol to his diet, and his wife exercising portion control—Neil's total cholesterol had fallen to 157. The 5-foot-5 retired civil engineer and former U.S. Army corporal had also lost 38 pounds, bringing his weight to 174. Says Neil, "I'm feeling very good about the changes I've made."

WINNING ACTION

Alter your meat-to-vegetables ratio. Eliminating meat from your diet is a good way to lower cholesterol, but it's a more drastic step than many people want to take. You can continue to eat meat if you choose lean cuts, trim all visible fat, and then use half (or less) the amount recipes call for. Make up the difference with assorted vegetables. You'll reduce your consumption of fat, cholesterol, and calories while upping fiber and vitamins. The best part? The flavor of your chili, stews, soups, and casseroles will be the same. Only your arteries will know the difference!

++

SHE REPLACED HIGH-FAT FAVORITES WITH LOW-FAT VERSIONS

On most days for lunch, Jessie Maurer used to eat a double cheeseburger with bacon and two large orders of fries at a fast-food restaurant. But when her cholesterol hit 299 in 1998, Jessie quickly learned the art of substitution, replacing all her high-fat favorites with low-fat alternatives.

Cheeseburgers became burgers made of portobello mushrooms or ground turkey. Omelettes were prepared with egg substitute. French fries were ditched in favor of baked potato wedges seasoned with olive oil and herbs. "I realized I could eat a lot of things," says Jessie, 54, of Emmaus, Pennsylvania. "I just had to eat them a different way."

Although she walks ¾ mile to work every day, Jessie had a weight problem for years. But she never gave much thought to her cholesterol levels until she went through menopause in 1998 and her doctor suggested she have them checked out. "When they saw my results, they told me I was a ticking time bomb," she recalls. "My doctor, who had had heart surgery himself, told me to cut out the fat. If changing my diet didn't work, he was going to put me on medications."

Eager to avoid taking drugs, Jessie went on a quest for low-fat substitutes. She was surprised to discover it was easier than crash dieting, which for Jessie had meant a week of eating nothing but plain tuna. "I had crash-dieted so many times and always felt deprived," she says. "This was so much easier because I wasn't really depriving myself; I was just eating a different way."

Initially, the hardest part was grocery shopping. "Before, I never looked at labels, and we'd just throw things in the cart," she says. "Now, I had to pull my glasses out and read everything." What was once a 20-minute trip to the supermarket turned into an hour, as she learned to read nutrition labels and weed out the foods high in fat, cholesterol, and saturated fat.

Her vigilance has paid off in a lower cholesterol level, which fell to 210 by December 2000. She has also lost more than 60 pounds, dropping from a high of 186 in 1998 to her current weight of 124 on her 5-foot-7 frame.

The only food she could not adequately replace was mayonnaise, which has meant giving up two of her old favorites: macaroni and potato salads. "That was hard at first," says Jessie, who used to make a big bowl of one or the other and eat it through the week. "Pasta salads with low-fat dressing just aren't the same. So every once in a while, I'll sneak a little taste."

WINNING ACTION

Replace your high-fat faves with lower-fat ones. Low-fat substitutes for cholesterol-raising ones are abundant. Use them! If you make chili with ground turkey instead of ground beef, you eat 27 percent less fat. If you substitute frozen chocolate yogurt for chocolate ice cream, you save another 45 percent fat. Peruse magazines, cookbooks, and the Internet for low-fat recipes of your favorite dishes. By making healthier versions of high-fat foods instead of banning them from your diet, you'll be less likely to feel deprived and more likely to stick with good eating habits.

+++

HE MADE A FAST BREAK
FROM FAST FOOD

In his job as a recreation and sports director, Glen Flood works closely with nutrition, heart, stroke, and diabetes organizations to promote active living and an awareness of healthy lifestyles.

But until recently, the 30-year-old found it much easier to talk the talk than to walk the walk. "I used to believe that if I exercised some, I'd be okay to eat fast food," says Glen, who lives in Charlottetown, Prince Edward Island. "I'd think I was hungry, snack way too much between meals, and eat a lot of burgers and fries, as well as deep-fried foods."

The "snack now, work out later" policy didn't fare well. "Exercise was way too often put on the back burner," says Glen. "I'd put it off until the next day because I was convinced that I could get fit later." By the winter of 1998, his total cholesterol reading was over 300, and his LDL level was 208.

Glen didn't pay much attention to his health until he and

his fiancée started attending seminars sponsored by a company that markets supplements. "The seminars had stats about people as young as I am having serious illness caused by high cholesterol," he says. "They also presented everyone with pamphlets that had information about heredity and how high cholesterol runs in families.

"I have a family history of high blood pressure, high cholesterol, and heart problems," Glen continues. "That was a good reason to start making life changes."

Even with the same busy work schedule, Glen says he now takes lunch to work with him instead of heading for his favorite fast-food haunts. "I do my best not to snack," he says, "and when I do snack, I make it apples, oranges, and other fruit."

Glen has also made a point of committing himself to regular exercise. Drawing on his experience as a recreation director, he has tried out various activities, from circuit training to basketball to soccer. "Over time," he says, "exercise has become fun again, and I no longer see it as a task."

Since 1999, the 5-foot-6 Canadian has lowered his total cholesterol to a much healthier 200 and his LDL to 134. He's also lost 20 pounds, bringing himself down to a trimmer 160 pounds. "My awareness and knowledge have improved 100 percent," says Glen. "The changes have not been easy, but they've been positive!"

WINNING ACTION

Break the fast-food habit. You probably realize fast food isn't good for you, but do you really know what you're getting at the takeout window? A quarter-pound burger with cheese and super size fries from McDonald's, for example, contain 59 grams of fat (18 grams of which are saturated). That's 90 percent of the total fat and saturated fat you should have in a day. One slice of a cheese stuffed-crust *pizza from Pizza Hut contains 10 grams of saturated fat—half the daily recommended amount. If your workplace doesn't have a cafeteria, bring a bagged lunch instead of going out to eat. And when you drive around town, carry fruit in the car so you can avoid the drive-thrus.*

++

FOODS HIGH IN WATER HELP KEEP HER CHOLESTEROL LOW

Every day, by the time dinner rolls around, Erin Pavlina has easily eaten more than 10 servings of fruits and vegetables, and absorbed a lot of water in the process. Not only is Erin a devout vegan, but she focuses on foods that are made up primarily of water—70 percent water or more, to be exact. Her high-water diet has helped her shave more than 200 points off her triglycerides and improved her cholesterol counts, too.

Erin, a 32-year-old Canoga Park, California, resident, got the idea to eat water-rich foods from *The American Vegetarian Cookbook from the Fit for Life Kitchen* by Marilyn Diamond. "It said that our bodies are 60 to 90 percent water," she says. "It just made sense to eat foods that contain a high percentage of water."

The first time Erin had her cholesterol tested, she was 18, and the results were not good: 303. "My sister and I were told that we had high cholesterol, but we were young and we didn't care," she recalls.

Then in 1997, at the age of 27, Erin received more startling news: While her cholesterol had dropped slightly to 293, her triglycerides were an alarmingly high 390. Shaken by the numbers, she tried to give up the fast food in her diet, which sometimes involved two Big Macs and french fries a day. The numbers didn't budge. She also tried exercising at a gym, going every day for 4 months straight. That failed, too.

She even tried going vegetarian for 9 months, to no avail.

Then her husband suggested they follow the advice in Diamond's book, switching to a stricter vegan diet and concentrating on foods that contain no less than 70 percent water. For the next 3 months, the couple started each day with a fruit plate or fruit smoothie, made with ingredients like bananas, plums, grapes, pineapple, and watermelon. Lunch consisted of veggie sandwiches and stir-fries made with zucchini, squash, cabbage, broccoli, and carrots. Dinner was largely grains and soy foods. "The goal was to get 5 to 10 servings of fruits and vegetables by dinnertime," she says.

In just 3 months, her water-rich vegan diet was showing results. While her total cholesterol showed a modest decline to 253, her overall profile improved dramatically. Her LDL dipped from 180 to 150, while her HDL rose from 21 to 71. What's more, her triglycerides plummeted to 144. Erin also shed 20 pounds from her 5-foot-9 frame, dropping to 160. Stomach pains, which doctors had suspected were irritable bowel syndrome, went away, too. "I used to take two Tums a day, and suddenly I didn't need them at all," she says.

Erin has continued with her water-rich vegan diet. She now runs two Web sites, one of which sells gift baskets filled with vegan sweets. She believes the vegan desserts account for her recent jump in total cholesterol to 289, admittedly a point of frustration. But the other figures remain the same as they were 3 months after she started on her water-rich vegan diet.

WINNING ACTION

Focus on eating foods dense in water. Some of the highest include broccoli, carrots, beets, oranges, apples, boiled potatoes, bananas, and corn. Many of the same fruits that are high in water content also help lower cholesterol and form the core of a low-fat diet. Half a grapefruit, for in-

*stance, is 91 percent water, while a medium apple is 84
percent water. Both are high in a soluble fiber called
pectin, which helps lower cholesterol. The majority of other
fruits are good sources of soluble fiber, too.*

+++

HE BULKED UP WITH FIBER—
AND BEAT CHOLESTEROL COLD

Terry Terfinko wasn't feeling his usual self. The Emmaus,
Pennsylvania, resident didn't have as much energy as he used
to, and he didn't feel as mentally sharp. Not only that, but he
was worried because his mother's side of the family had heart
and cholesterol problems. So he went for a checkup.

At the doctor's office, Terry's fears were realized: His cholesterol was 213, his triglycerides 346. At 234 pounds, he
was 50 pounds over his high school weight. And to top it all
off, he had high blood pressure.

Terry knew that he had to change his habits; his days of
eating greasy cheesesteaks and fries were over. He read up on
nutrition and learned that eating high-fiber meals would keep
him fuller longer, so he could eat less and still not feel deprived. "I started eating more fruits and vegetables. And I
came to like seven-grain cereals," Terry says. "I make a mix
of psyllium and oat bran and sprinkle it on cereal. I even put
it in bread and pancakes. Eating more fiber makes my stomach feel full."

Switching to high-fiber foods wasn't hard for Terry. It was
just a matter of making some clever substitutions, such as
whole wheat bread for white and high-fiber cereal in place of
regular. And he didn't even miss the high-fat, high-calorie
foods he cut out. "When I eat those old foods now, it doesn't
feel good," he says. "It got so that I came to prefer foods in
their natural state—a potato instead of french fries or potato
chips, whole fresh fruit instead of canned."

Besides going the high-fiber route, Terry became a biking devotee, increasing his endurance until he was cycling over 5,000 miles per year.

It worked. By 1998, 2 years after his initial diagnosis, Terry learned that his cholesterol was down to 143 and his triglycerides had dropped to 90. "My doctor was amazed at the results," he says. "I went off the blood pressure meds. My weight is currently 182 pounds, and at age 48, I have the energy of a 20-year-old."

WINNING ACTION

Reach for high-fiber foods. Make it your mission to find sneaky but simple ways to get more fiber into your diet. You'll feel full while eating less food. And the fiber itself can actually help lower your cholesterol. Read labels carefully so you can replace low-fiber breads and cereals with their high-fiber counterparts. Sprinkle wheat germ, psyllium, and oat bran on cereal, yogurt, and ice cream. Or use them to replace some of the flour in homemade pancakes and bread.

++

A BIG DIET CHANGE GAVE HIM BIG RESULTS

Charles Wilkes does not hesitate when asked what he did to cut his cholesterol level. "I became a vegan," he says. "I eat no animal products, not even dairy."

And the explanation for his success is simple: "Cholesterol totally comes from animal products," he says. "Cut them out, and you cut out cholesterol."

Charles, a 75-year-old IBM retiree who lives in San Jose, California, was diagnosed with adult-onset (type 2) diabetes in 1998. "That was a shock to me; you know that they call diabetes the silent killer," he says. "I knew that something had to change."

Along with high blood sugar levels, Charles also had high cholesterol. "It was about 260, which the doctors at that time called marginal," he says. "They told me that I had the right ratio [of total cholesterol to HDL], so it wasn't a concern."

Still, Charles wasn't going to take any chances with his health. He says that he "bought just about every book available" on diet and its effects on diabetes. And the more he read, the more he came to believe that the dietary changes he would make to control his blood sugar would help get his cholesterol down, too.

"I was pretty ignorant," he says. "I like cottage cheese, and I always ate it for breakfast. I thought of it kind of like a salad. But it was full-fat, which didn't help my cholesterol at all. Now I start my day with grapefruit. And I don't miss the cottage cheese at all."

Also gone from Charles's diet were eggs, milk, and other dairy products, as well as meat. "Had I known before what I know now, I would never have eaten meat at all," he says.

Within 4 months, when he returned to his doctor, Charles was told that the results he had achieved were "awesome." Today, his cholesterol is 150, with LDL of 66 and HDL of 39. His triglycerides are down to 223.

As an added benefit, Charles's blood sugar level dropped enough that he was able to cut his dosage of medicine in half. Now his blood sugar measures between 80 and 120 milligrams of plasma glucose per deciliter of blood.

Charles says that he tries to eat as many raw fruits and vegetables as possible. He eats a lot of tomatoes and drinks carrot juice. He also takes Barleygreen, a powder made from the juice of young sprigs of barley. "I am never hungry," he says.

His next challenge is getting his wife, Alice, 16 years his junior and a native of the Philippines, to improve her diet.

"She eats a lot of meat," he says. But he is not tempted, even when he smells what she is eating. "I don't remember smelling anything that makes me want to break my diet," he says. "I really support the lifestyle I'm in."

WINNING ACTION

Adopt a vegan diet. It won't appeal to everyone, but a vegan diet—which allows only plant foods and no animal products—can help rein in high cholesterol. That's because meats and dairy are leading sources of saturated fat and cholesterol in the typical diet. On the other hand, a low-fat, low-cholesterol diet—which describes veganism to a tee—is the best way to reduce elevated blood cholesterol without medication. Plenty of fruits, vegetables, beans, and whole grains are the key to success.

Note: The American Diabetes Association recommends that people with high cholesterol be routinely screened for diabetes. People with diabetes have a greater risk of developing heart disease and hardening of the arteries than those without diabetes.

+++

SAVORY INGREDIENTS MAKE HER FORGET ABOUT MEAT

Life without meat? Years ago, Susan Bass would have thought it inconceivable. "I truly loved meat. I ate it every single day," says the 56-year-old retired special education teacher from Flossmoor, Illinois. "I collected reams of recipes with meat as an ingredient."

Today, those recipes sit yellowing in a kitchen drawer. Susan hasn't taken so much as a bite of steak since 1997. The former meat-lover favors meatless meals that get their flavor not from fat but from unique, zesty condiments and season-ings.

What brought about Susan's change of heart? A massive heart attack in August 1996, followed by a year of trying to rein in her dangerously high cholesterol, which had climbed to an astounding 400. "As I recall, my LDL was around 200, and my HDL was about 20," she says. "My overall profile could not have been much worse."

Realizing the seriousness of her situation, Susan immediately snuffed out her 20-year, two-pack-a-day smoking habit. Surprisingly, that wasn't her greatest challenge. "It was much easier than giving up meat," she admits.

At first, Susan followed the American Heart Association diet, which permitted occasional servings of lean beef and poultry. Her cholesterol—which was being tested monthly—didn't budge. Even cholesterol-lowering drugs didn't help. "I felt like I was another heart attack waiting to happen," she says.

Then Susan's doctor recommended that she enroll in the Rice Diet Program at Duke University in Durham, North Carolina. Susan stayed at the clinic for 2½ months, attending classes in nutrition and cooking, exercise, and meditation. In addition, she was put on a very low fat, low-sodium diet featuring plenty of rice, fruit, and steamed vegetables.

"In just 3 weeks, my cholesterol dropped dramatically. When I left the clinic, it was down to 170," Susan says. "When I saw the numbers, I knew that diet had done the trick."

Once she left the clinic, Susan vowed to stick with her newly reformed eating habits. A passionate cook, she invested in cookbooks featuring fat-free, low-sodium meatless recipes and browsed specialty shops for interesting, healthy condiments and seasonings. "You can make very tasty dishes, even with no fat and very little salt," she says. "For example, I serve my sea bass with a wonderful roasted garlic and onion jam from a company called Stonewall Kitchen.

And I found a great no-salt mustard that I mix into tuna salad instead of mayonnaise."

Susan also spritzes balsamic vinegar on her salads, drizzles Hunt's No Salt Added Ketchup on her baked potatoes, and stuffs squash into her ravioli. Even her breakfast cereal gets special treatment. "Fat-free milk is off-limits, so I pour pineapple juice over my puffed wheat," she says. "I think it tastes great!"

Susan's savvy use of condiments and seasonings has kept her loyal to her heart-healthy diet. That—combined with a regular walking regimen and cholesterol-lowering medication—has improved Susan's cholesterol profile even more. Her latest test results are nothing less than impressive: total cholesterol of 145, with her LDL at 67 and her HDL at 58.

While Susan has worked hard to achieve those numbers, she doesn't take all of the credit. "I truly believe the only reason I am here is because of the Rice Diet Program," she says. "The doctors were wonderful. They saved my life!"

WINNING ACTION

Expand your flavor repertoire. There's no denying that fat makes food taste good. But eaten in excess, it can drive cholesterol to a dangerously high level. That said, cutting your fat intake doesn't have to mean giving up flavor. These days, you can buy all sorts of condiments and seasonings that add fat-free zest to your favorite recipes. Your supermarket probably has an array of products from which to choose—but don't forget to check out health food stores and specialty stores as well. Remember, too, that certain herbs and spices—like garlic and turmeric— contain compounds that help lower cholesterol. What a wonderful bonus!

SHE COULDN'T GIVE UP THE BAKERY, SO SHE STARTED HER OWN

Allison Rivers has an unabashed sweet tooth, which has meant a lifetime of eating cookies, muffins, and just about anything else sweet. But at 18, when she learned she had high cholesterol, she began looking for ways to make her cherished baked goods without cholesterol.

Allison, a 31-year-old resident of Agoura Hills, California, first found out about her cholesterol problem more than 12 years ago, when a blood test performed at her health club showed her total cholesterol to be 212. "It totally freaked me out," she recalls. "Everyone on my mom's side of the family is obese, and most of them died of heart problems. So I thought, wow, if this is what my genetic situation is, then I need to make some changes now."

After a doctor confirmed the results of her first test, Allison started taking an over-the-counter niacin supplement to lower her cholesterol. But the niacin made her itchy and flushed, a common side effect, so she quit. A newly confirmed vegetarian, Allison decided to try going vegan—meaning she'd eat no animal products. She increased the amount of fruits and vegetables in her diet, switched from white rice to brown rice, and opted for chocolate soy ice cream over the mint cookie or coffee ice cream she used to love.

But finding tasty baked goods was another matter for Allison, who had a habit of starting her mornings with a "gooey cinnamon roll." She tried vegan products but thought they tasted awful. So she decided to take matters into her own hands and changed the way she baked. She replaced eggs with a powdered egg substitute made of potato starch and baking powder. She ditched the butter in favor of sunflower oil. And instead of milk, she used soy or rice milk. "I have an incredible sweet tooth, so giving up sweets was not an option," she says. "That's why I started playing with these recipes."

Allison, who was then working in retail, shared her newly concocted recipes with her colleagues, who sang their praises. At their urging, she began selling her baked goods (cookies and brownies) on the Internet. Today, she runs her own business, Allison's Gourmet, which features vegan baked goods.

For more than a decade, Allison avoided getting her cholesterol tested. But a recent test showed that her total cholesterol had dropped to 126. She has also taken up walking and hiking and feels less stress these days from owning her own business and being her own boss. Best of all, she's managed to take control of her cholesterol without sacrificing her favorite sweets.

WINNING ACTION

Try cutting fat and cholesterol in the baked goods you make. Eggs, butter, sour cream, and whole milk, for instance, can all be replaced with healthier alternatives. As a vegan, Allison doesn't use dairy products. But you can try fat-free egg substitute, nonfat sour cream, canola oil, and fat-free milk. You can even replace some of the fat in baked goods with applesauce or prune puree. In the process, you'll cut back on not only cholesterol but also saturated fat, one of the prime dietary culprits for raising cholesterol.

++

HE LETS THE CHEESE STAND ALONE

Ed Hoey is a fan of cheese: cheese sandwiches, macaroni and cheese, crackers and cheese. "All variations of cheese—I love them," he says.

But he also has high cholesterol. And cheese, except for

low-fat and nonfat varieties, is high in cholesterol-producing fat. Many hard cheeses derive more than half their calories from fat—and that's saturated fat, which the American Heart Association recommends should make up less than 10 percent of daily calories.

So Ed had to do something. Despite the fact that he was eating "lots of fruits and vegetables" and doing lots of walking, snowshoeing, and golfing, his cholesterol was up to 300.

In 1999, his doctor gave him a prescription for Lipitor. He also recommended that Ed, then 73, cut back on cheese.

Ed followed his doctor's orders. Within 4 months, his cholesterol had dropped to 200. The doctor lowered his dosage of Lipitor from 10 milligrams a day to 10 milligrams every other day. Now he's down to 5 milligrams every other day. His cholesterol level remains at 200.

And he still enjoys an occasional bite of cheese.

"I used to have cheese three or four times a week," says Ed, of Syracuse, New York. "Now I have it just once every couple of weeks." Like the occasional bowl of ice cream he allows himself, cheese is a treat, he says. Thinking of it as a rare pleasure to be savored has helped him to limit how much of it he eats.

Ed says that reducing the amount of cheese in his diet was not difficult. "My motivation was that 300 cholesterol reading," he says. "I just decided to do it, and I did it."

WINNING ACTION

Think of cheese as a treat. A cholesterol-lowering diet has little room for big quantities of high-fat cheese. But considering that Americans eat three times as much cheese today as they did in 1970 (more than 8 billion pounds a year), it's a craving many people find hard to deny. So don't deny it. Instead, put it in the same "treat" category you reserve for birthday cakes, buttered popcorn at the movies, and Easter candy. When you do eat cheese, give it your full attention and savor it. Absentmindedly noshing it won't satisfy your craving and will lead to overeating it. Of course, if you learn to love nonfat varieties, you can indulge more often.

+++

SHE CUT OUT DAIRY AND BEAT TWO DISEASES AT ONCE

In 1995, Sabrina Nelson's cholesterol was 265. But her doctors weren't concerned with that, because the 35-year-old resident of Los Angeles had a much more pressing illness: relapsing polychondritis, an autoimmune disease that causes the body to become allergic to itself and start attacking cartilage.

Hoping to find a way to stall the illness, Sabrina studied nutrition books and discovered a possible link between dairy and autoimmune disease. Already a vegetarian, she decided to go one step further and eliminate dairy products from her diet. Out went the ice cream, the cheese, and the milk, and in came the tofu ice cream, soy cheese, and the rice milk.

Besides nixing the dairy, Sabrina began an exercise program, so her body would have the strength to heal itself. She also took up cross-stitching, which helps her relax when she's stressed.

A mere 3 months after cutting dairy from her diet, Sabrina's relapsing polychondritis was in complete remission. And as a bonus, her cholesterol had dropped from 265 all the way down to 135.

Were there any times when Sabrina just wanted to indulge in an ice cream sundae or a slice of cheese pizza? "I just remember how much healthier I feel without that bowl of ice cream or glass of milk," she says firmly. Making the decision even easier was the plethora of delicious dairy substitutes on the market. "As soy products are so wonderful these days, giving up dairy is no sacrifice."

Not only did Sabrina discover that dairy substitutes fit the bill, but she also found a whole world of scrumptious dairy-free dishes from Chinese, Indian, Thai, Vietnamese, and other cuisines. "I discovered hundreds of foods," she says. "I consider the way I eat an adventure."

Sabrina believes that her dairy-free lifestyle will bring her health and happiness. "I've been blessed; that is truly the way I feel," she says. "I wish other people could be as lucky as I am."

WINNING ACTION

Rethink your choices from the dairy case. Many people rely on milk and other dairy products for their daily dose of calcium. These foods are top-notch sources of the mineral, but the full-fat versions are high in cholesterol-raising saturated fat. While you don't need to give up dairy completely, as Sabrina did, your best bet is to stick with low-fat and fat-free versions of your favorite products. You can also try low-fat or fat-free dairy substitutes like soy milk, rice milk, almond milk, soy cheese, and soy sour cream.

Keep in mind, too, that other foods contain impressive amounts of calcium. Good sources include canned salmon and sardines with bones, almonds, figs, and Chinese cabbage (bok choy).

++

HE WHETS—AND WETS—HIS SWEET TOOTH WITH ICE POPS

Howard Goldberg has a wicked sweet tooth. It was cultivated early on by his mother, who spent her days baking pies and cakes and making fudge. So when it came time to lower his cholesterol, Howard knew he'd have to tame his sugar cravings. He found his answer in the grocer's freezer.

These days, when his sweet tooth beckons, Howard indulges in frozen pops—cherry, grape, or orange with no fat, cholesterol, sugar, or sodium. He buys two boxes a week at a price of $3 for 15 bars. Some nights, when the urge is especially strong, he eats two at a time. "They're really wonderful," he says.

Howard, 57, of Springfield, Massachusetts, grew up in a home where dessert was as certain as the sunrise. "No meal was complete unless you had dessert," he says. "I love sweets. I could eat a pound of fudge." Indeed, Howard indulged in "anything that looked sticky, gooey, and delicious," which included cakes, pies, and chocolate—all full of fat as well as sugar.

In 1999, his cholesterol hit 220. "When I found out I had high cholesterol, I knew I had to cut back on my desserts," he says. That's when he became stricter with his diet. Eventually, he cut back on sweets in favor of more fresh salads and fruits.

Desserts became a rare treat, reserved for special occasions, such as having dinner guests. Even then, any leftover goodies go home with the visitors. And instead of the fat-laden sweets he used to love, Howard is content with berries and melons, sometimes topped with Cool Whip.

As his appetite for desserts diminished, so did his cholesterol count. After about 6 months, his cholesterol bottomed out at 180, where it still hovers. At the same time, his weight dropped from 245 pounds to 210. Although he's gained a little of that back, at 6 feet 2 inches, he's holding steady at 225 pounds.

Howard says he has to allow himself the occasional treat if he's to survive the self-imposed restrictions on dessert. But it's the ice pops that get him through the day-to-day cravings for something sweet. "Nothing replaces chocolate, but if we're sitting around watching TV or reading and want something sweet, these make a great guilt-free snack," he says.

WINNING ACTION

Eat nonfat, sugar-free ice pops and other sweet treats. There's more than sugar in the desserts most people crave. The fat and cholesterol that generally keep sugar company pack on the pounds and raise your body's cholesterol levels. Low-fat, low-sugar (or sugar-free) desserts can be equally satisfying. You just have to give your tastebuds a chance to adjust to them. Besides ice pops, try no-sugar sweets like pudding made with fat-free milk, or nonfat yogurt and ice cream. Gussy them up with luscious ripe berries or other fruit. Remember that although angel food cake and meringues do contain sugar, they have no fat or cholesterol and are lower in calories than most other desserts.

++

SHE SCRAPPED THE SCRAPPLE— AND HER CHOLESTEROL

When you work around food for a living, you're constantly tempted to help polish off anything left over at the end of the day. Marie Schollenberger, 65, of Boyertown, Pennsylvania, found that out the hard way.

In addition to waitressing for a catering service 3 or 4 days a week, Marie also helps out at a firehouse—and working at a firehouse invariably entails eating there. "They serve a nice Sunday breakfast, and we get to have what's left," she says.

What's left is invariably a cholesterol nightmare: sausage, eggs, and scrapple, a Pennsylvania specialty made from cornmeal and ground pork or sausage that's sliced and fried. Each serving of scrapple can contain a good amount of saturated fat. "It's hard to pick good things to eat there because everything is fried," says Marie.

In 2000, though, Marie realized that she had to reform her ways. Her total cholesterol level stood at 300, and her physician said that she had to either lower her numbers or take medication. "I didn't want to go on medication because I'm taking medication for other things," she says.

Marie's workplace proved the ideal spot to reform her past eating habits. She dropped the sausage, eggs, and scrapple and started looking for healthier alternatives. Since she had access to the kitchen, she was able to make salads for herself. She brought in egg substitute for use in her own meals. She started ordering the baked haddock and refrained from putting any butter on it.

She also took to walking the country roads near her house three times a week, a mile at a time. She plans to buy weights to make the walks even more effective.

Marie's yearlong efforts brought her total cholesterol down to 231, with an LDL level of 145. She is working to get the numbers even lower. "A lot of people who eat where I work are taking cholesterol-lowering medicine," she says, but they use it as an excuse to have whatever they want. "Even if they order Egg Beaters, they get the scrapple and fried potatoes as well. I can't tell them what to eat; they're my customers."

WINNING ACTION

Don't let where you work dictate what you eat. It's always easier to go with what's available, whether it's the scrapple on the griddle or the candy bars in the vending machine. But every time you settle for what's easy, your body "settles" in as well. Do yourself a favor and take your own lunch or snacks to munch on during the day.

++

SHE ZONED IN ON BALANCE

In 1991, Penny Tennant was diagnosed with polycystic ovaries, a painful condition that some researchers believe is related to the body's improper use of insulin. For help, Penny turned to a diet that others with the same condition have used to lower insulin levels. And in the process, she got her cholesterol under control.

"I was really surprised," says Penny, 39, of Sunnyvale, California. "I thought I had been doing all the things that were right. But the new diet made a difference."

The diet Penny is referring to is the Zone, popularized by Barry Sears, Ph.D. Before she started it, her cholesterol reading was 250. Two months later, it was down to 173, with a ratio (a comparison of total cholesterol to HDL) of 2 and triglycerides of 73.

As a bonus, Penny shed some unwanted pounds. At 5 feet 8 inches, she used to weigh 144. Now she's down to 134. And while she still has pain from her polycystic ovaries, it's not nearly as severe.

The Zone diet is based on a constant balance of fats, carbohydrates, and proteins. Each meal, including midafternoon and evening snacks, consists of 30 percent fat, 30 percent protein, and 40 percent carbohydrates. The carbohydrates, Penny says, are "good carbs"—salad, broccoli, whole grain breads. Potatoes, carrots, and bananas are limited because of their sugar content.

"On this program, you always eat good fats with every meal," she adds. Good fats—meaning monounsaturates—are found in foods such as olive oil, canola oil, avocados, and nuts. Researchers believe they may actually lower LDL levels without negatively affecting HDL cholesterol to the extent that a diet higher in carbohydrates and lower in fat could.

Penny says that she drinks a lot of water during the day. "Sometimes, you think you are hungry, and really you are just thirsty," she notes.

She also tries to exercise, doing brisk walking and moderate weight lifting whenever she has a chance. "But I've got small children," she says. "I do my best."

The Zone diet permits consumption of soft and low-fat cheeses, as well as small amounts of ice cream ("the real stuff," Penny says). Fatty meats and eggs are discouraged, and hydrogenated oils are eliminated.

Although Penny finds following the diet expensive, she says it's worth the cost. "It makes me feel good," she says. "I am really even-tempered, and I have good energy. If I eat lunch at McDonald's or Denny's, I don't get anything done all afternoon. But if I have a Zone lunch, I feel wonderful. I get a lot done, and I'm not sleepy."

WINNING ACTION

Balance proteins, carbohydrates, and fats. The Zone diet works for many people, but it's not for everybody. The American Heart Association recommends a more moderate approach: about 15 percent protein, 55 percent or more carbs, and 30 percent or less fat. Because it's difficult for most people to make these calculations, try this approach to meals: Mentally divide your plate into quarters. Allocate one-quarter for lean protein, one-half for vegetables or fruits, and one-quarter for whole grains. You'll get plenty of cholesterol-lowering fiber without an overload of fat, especially saturated fat.

++

HE CUT BACK ON JUNK FOOD AND REGAINED HIS HEALTH

William Caldwell was near death. When attacks of unstable angina roused him during the night, a fourth-year medical student sleeping in the hospital room across from his was there in an instant. The doctor-to-be guided the nurses with their ministrations of medicine and calmed William, lest tension make the angina worse.

At age 65, William, of Kokomo, Indiana, had developed heart blockages so severe that he couldn't walk to his mailbox. He underwent a cardiac catheterization to diagnose the problem, two angioplasty procedures to unclog the arteries, and, when those same arteries were closed again within 2 months, a triple coronary bypass.

Two months later, he was back in the hospital after having a heart attack.

"My body must grow a lot of scar tissue," says William. "All three bypass grafts were closed off in a couple of months due to scar tissue."

His doctors wanted to perform another bypass operation. "But they couldn't guarantee that it would work," William says. "The surgeons promised me 7 good years 'if' they were successful. I told them that I didn't like the word 'if' and that I wanted to try another method."

His doctors were adamant. They told him he shouldn't leave the hospital; when he insisted, the cardiologists considered dropping him as a patient. In the end, William won. "They reluctantly dismissed me," he says. "They said they would continue to treat me but they didn't agree with what I was doing. They told my wife that my chances of living without surgery were very slim."

Once home, William drastically changed his diet. He eliminated all junk food. "You wouldn't believe what I used to eat: cakes, pies, doughnuts," he says. "I would take stuff to work with me and then get more food from the vending machines." He also cut out beef, which was something he had eaten nearly every day all his life.

He substituted fruits, vegetables, and whole grains for his former unhealthy staples. Four months after he returned home—and just a week before he was scheduled for another bypass operation, something he had agreed to when his progress seemed so slow—his wife looked at him over the breakfast table. "Are you feeling better today?" she asked.

"Yes, I am," William responded. "Why do you ask?"

"Because your color is back."

William canceled the bypass surgery. Ten years later, he walks up to 2 miles a day. He swims twice a week and exercises at the gym three times a week. His total cholesterol, 245 at its highest, is down to 180. His cholesterol ratio (a comparison of total cholesterol to HDL) is 3 to 1; it had been 6 to 1. Triglycerides that had been up to 600 are at 150.

"I feel great," he says. "I know that I made the right decision. I was afraid that scar tissue would again prematurely close the bypasses, and I would be gone."

William still eats no cholesterol-raising hydrogenated or partially hydrogenated oils, instead enjoying whole grains, fruits, and vegetables. When eggs are called for, he uses egg substitute, and all cheese on his dinner table is fat-free. Recently, he added salmon, soy milk, soy veggie burgers, and soy margarine to his diet, along with flaxseed oil. "I am still tweaking my diet," he says. "I never eat more than 10 grams of saturated fat or more than 100 milligrams of cholesterol per day."

"I made a drastic change," he adds. "But I was desperate. I love life and wanted to live. A lot of people can't do what I have done. They can't give up foods they have eaten all their lives. But maybe they just aren't motivated the way I was."

WINNING ACTION

Cut out junk foods, even if it means a drastic change in your diet. Junk foods offer little that's good to your body and lots that's bad. They're high in fat (especially saturated fat), cholesterol, sugar, salt, or calories—and they usually contain a combination of these elements that drive up your risk of high cholesterol. Trading them in for fruits, vegetables, whole grain foods, and lean meats will go a long way toward bringing down your cholesterol. But you don't have to give up "fun foods," especially if they enhance your enjoyment of life. Just make smarter choices. Look for fat-free baked goods, low-sodium chips and other snacks, and low-cal ice cream and candies. Make nachos with fat-free cheese and no-cholesterol sour cream and refried beans. Your tastebuds won't know the difference, but your body will.

++

HE FOUND THE PERFECT "NO-DIET" DIET

When Richard Chernela learned in 1999 that his total cholesterol level was 214, he knew that it was a bit high. But he didn't worry about it.

He had bigger problems, after all, thanks to a triglyceride level that practically broke the scales at 476. "With my triglycerides so high, I realized that I was at risk," says the 51-year-old resident of South Orange, New Jersey. "Lowering my cholesterol was secondary; my primary goal was to bring my triglyceride level down."

His doctor suggested taking a statin drug to improve the cholesterol readings, but Richard first wanted to see what he could accomplish without resorting to drugs. "I felt that having to take medication to reduce my triglyceride level was some kind of failure on my part to control what I believed was controllable," he says.

Richard leapt into action. Within just 4 months, his total cholesterol decreased to 185, his HDL level increased from 22 to 47, and his triglyceride level dropped all the way to 99.

What was his secret? Did he find some great new fad diet that helped the pounds and cholesterol melt away?

Just the opposite, in fact. Richard credits his astounding success to shunning fad diets in favor of the basics of sensible weight and cholesterol reduction: eating less and exercising more. "Getting hung up on the particulars of a strict regimen or going on an Atkins or Zone diet just makes it too complicated," he says. "And unless that diet restricts the number of calories coming in, it just ain't going to work. Besides, who the devil wants to spend the rest of his life adhering to those diets? The important thing is that reducing calorie intake is a permanent dietary change, not a temporary quick fix."

Some of the smart, simple moves Richard made include replacing his morning buttered bagel with whole grain cereal and a banana; decreasing the portion size of meats, fish, and poultry in his meals; and reducing desserts from a daily fact of life to a once-weekly event.

Of course, being an adherent of the tried-and-true health basics, Richard also added exercise to the mix. He began running, starting slowly and increasing the intensity of his workouts until eventually he ran a 5K race at an 8:15-per-mile pace.

Besides losing 20 pounds and reducing his cholesterol, Richard sleeps less and has more energy. "I feel great," he says. "I still get a kick out of putting on clothes I used to wear and seeing how baggy they are on me."

WINNING ACTION

Avoid fad diets. Trying out every new diet that comes down the pike can be complicated and discouraging. Instead of counting calories, weighing food, or drastically reducing certain food groups, consider the old standby weight-loss method that has worked for generations: Eat less than you did in the past, and start moving!

++

SHE OUTGREW THE FOODS
OF HER CHILDHOOD

LaVonnia Johnson grew up with a cook in the house. "It was my father, and we ate well," recalls the 50-year-old Greensboro, North Carolina, native. "We had butter, eggs, fried chicken, fried fish, apple pies, pumpkin pies, and parfaits."

And for breakfast? "My father would wake us up and say, 'What do you want?' " LaVonnia says. "Whatever it was, he would fix it for us—pancakes, French toast, scrambled eggs, bacon."

These days, breakfast means brown rice cereal or oatmeal to LaVonnia. Fried foods are out, and sweets—well, LaVonnia is still working on eliminating them from her diet. But she is doing pretty well at following her doctor's orders, issued around 1995, to get her diet "under control." While she doesn't mention the specific numbers, her cholesterol profile has improved considerably. As a bonus, her dress size went from 22 to 14 after she lost 55 pounds. At 5 feet 5½ inches, she weighs 170 pounds.

"I had to completely reevaluate how I eat," she says. The traditional African-American foods that she grew up with are gone or at least modified. "I've learned to use olive oil and to throw away the fat from meats," she says. "Most Black people save the fat to use later."

She has eliminated beef from her diet and is "trying to get rid of chicken." She has cut her bread intake from two or three pieces to one a day, has boosted the amount of heart-healthy sardines and salmon she eats, and no longer stops off for fast-food meals. Added to her diet is garlic—five cloves a week, cut up finely and swallowed with water. "Only when I chew it up do I get a garlic smell," she says.

But LaVonnia did not stop with her diet. A congressional staff assistant, LaVonnia exercises at the gym 3 hours a day, 2 in the morning and 1 in the evening.

The first part of her morning routine is a cardiac fitness

workout. She spends 30 minutes on a step machine and 25 minutes on either a treadmill or a bicycle. That is followed by 30 minutes of weight lifting and 25 minutes of exercise intended to strengthen abdominal muscles. "Sometimes, I do 500 crunches," she says.

Her evening exercise used to consist of swimming. After a bout of ear infections, she now alternates among the treadmill, stretches, and abdominal work.

LaVonnia says she feels great. She has convinced her children to follow her example. As for her father, the great cook of her childhood, he is 80 and still lives in Greensboro. Primrose Perkins followed the advice of his own doctor and now "he eats better than I do," says LaVonnia.

"I feel blessed," she adds. "We are all healthier because our doctors convinced us to take a look at our diets."

WINNING ACTION

Don't be bound by the traditional foods of your childhood. It is easy to slip into patterns that were established at your parents' dinner table, but it is not always healthy to do so. Keep in mind that many ethnic foods can be modified to reduce fats while keeping the basic flavor you love. Traditional African-American foods such as greens and sweet potatoes, for example, are rich in vitamins and fiber and are delicious without bacon fat or butter. With substitutions of canola oil for butter and whole wheat for white flour, even pancakes can become cholesterol busters.

+++

HE STARTS HIS MEALS OFF RIGHT

Beef fajitas. Fried chicken. Ice cream and cinnamon rolls. These were the standards of John Houck's diet. But when his doctor ordered him to get his cholesterol down or go on medication, John adjusted. Now, 13 pounds lighter and with a much healthier cholesterol level, he indulges in fatty foods only occasionally. And when he does, he has a surefire strategy for making sure he doesn't go overboard.

"I try to start each meal with a substantial serving of vegetables," says John. "That way, I get a lot of vegetables, and I am not all that hungry for other things when I am done."

By "substantial serving," John means an entire bell pepper. A giant carrot. A stalk of broccoli. A quarter head of cauliflower. Even an entire bunch of spinach. "And I try to eat it raw whenever I can," says John, who's 41 and lives in Austin, Texas.

John was diagnosed with a cholesterol problem in September 1999. His total cholesterol was 217, with an LDL of 154. "The doctor said that with my family history, I had to either get it down or go on medicine," says John. "There was no way I was doing that. I am not a big fan of medicines."

John's maternal grandmother had a heart attack when she was in her forties. Her sons, John's father and uncle, were both 50 when they died of heart attacks. John's cousin, son of the uncle, had Marfan's syndrome, which weakened his heart muscle. He had to undergo open-heart surgery at age 18 and died on the operating table.

So John understood the importance of taking care of himself. Immediately, he reduced his meat consumption by more than half. He also gave up fajitas and fried chicken in favor of more vegetables.

As for exercise, John—a former world champion in freestyle Frisbee—got a good workout playing Ultimate, a soccerlike game that uses a flying disc instead of a ball. John also designs and installs courses for disc golf, which is similar to regular golf, except that it's played with a flying disc rather than with a golf club and ball.

Three months after John's initial diagnosis, his cholesterol was down to 180, and his weight had dropped from 189 to

176 (John is 5 feet 5). "I relaxed my diet a bit after receiving the good news, and my cholesterol still went down even more," he says. At his last reading, his cholesterol was 161, with an LDL of 99. His weight held steady.

Now, John eats fajitas or fried chicken about once a week, pizza once in a while. But the cinnamon rolls, something he developed a fondness for in 1993 when his kitchen was out of commission for a couple of weeks, are on the "rare list."

"I ran the other day, and I told myself that when I finished, I could get myself a cinnamon roll," he says. "But I fought off the craving. I had a low-fat yogurt instead. It was good enough."

WINNING ACTION

Start each meal with a large helping of vegetables. It's a great way to satisfy your immediate hunger and can prevent you from overindulging in other foods that are higher in fat and cholesterol. Further, vegetables contain no cholesterol and barely any fat (as long as they aren't adorned with butter or cheese). The fiber in vegetables is a proven cholesterol reducer, and vegetables are high in essential nutrients like vitamins A and C, folate, iron, and magnesium. Strive to get at least three to five servings a day.

++

CUTTING OUT ADDED OILS TOOK HIM ALL THE WAY TO HIS GOAL

Eric Fricker tried everything he could think of. He became a vegetarian, eliminating all animal products, including dairy foods. He drank soy lecithin shakes. And still his cholesterol, at 180, was higher than he wanted.

"I was not satisfied," he says. "I was reading information

from the Physicians Committee for Responsible Medicine, and I knew that a cholesterol level of 150 is best for preventing cardiovascular disease. That is what I kept trying to get to."

The Internet site for the Physicians Committee (www.pcrm.org) quotes information from the Framingham Heart Study, in which residents of Framingham, Massachusetts, and their rates of heart disease have been monitored since 1948. The study, now under the direction of Daniel Levy, M.D., has shown that the ideal cholesterol level "appears to be below 150 mg/dL. At that point, a heart attack is very unlikely."

So Eric took an additional step. He eliminated all added oils—oils that did not appear naturally in the fruits, vegetables, and whole grains he was eating. Finally, his cholesterol level dropped to 145. His ratio of total cholesterol to HDL dropped to 3.37 from a high of 9, and his triglycerides went from 505 to 157.

Since then, he has experimented with his diet to determine whether those oils really did make a difference. "I added oils back in, and my cholesterol went back up to 180," he says.

Eric, who's 40 and lives in Cocoa Beach, Florida, is a civilian software engineer on an air force base. He first learned that his cholesterol was high during a general screening at work in 1993. "It was 242, so I figured I'd better start doing something," he says. The soy lecithin reduced his level to 220, and he was just deciding what to try next when his wife announced that the family—including three children, ages 3, 5, and 7—was going vegetarian. A month later, they were all vegans, eating no animal products at all, not even dairy foods.

Eric's diet has had benefits other than lowered cholesterol. He has gone from 183 pounds to 165 and has lost that "spare tire" he was sporting.

What's more, his energy level has increased. "I was a real couch potato, always sitting around watching TV," he says. "I now surf two or three times a week."

Making changes was not always easy for Eric. "Cheese took me about 2 months to get over, and added fat about a month to get over," he says. "But we are leaving a legacy for our family. We did this as a team effort so that we wouldn't have health problems and pass them on to our children."

WINNING ACTION

Give up added oils. Oil adds calories to food (120 calories per tablespoon), and added calories can mean weight gain, a significant factor in heart disease risk and elevated cholesterol. If completely giving up oils is too drastic a step for you, cut back on your overall consumption and reach for those oils high in monounsaturated fat (such as olive and canola). There's evidence that monounsaturates can lower total blood cholesterol while increasing good HDL cholesterol. Note: Experts advise against getting less than 10 percent of total calories from fat.

++

SHE SATISFIED HER CHOCOLATE CRAVINGS WITH TOOTSIE ROLLS

Mikki Smoak knows about heart trouble. She was born with aortic stenosis, a condition in which the opening of the aortic valve is narrow, forcing the heart to pump harder than normal. After two major surgeries to correct the condition, Mikki was frustrated to learn that she had a cholesterol problem. She was ready to do anything to stay heart healthy—even give up her beloved chocolate.

But rather than abandon the taste of chocolate altogether, Mikki took up eating Tootsie Rolls—lots of them. She shops in a giant warehouse, where she buys 5-pound bags of the little candies, then stashes handfuls of them in her purse, desk, bookbag, and car. "Tootsie Rolls really do help me," says Mikki, a 52-year-old college student from Charleston, South Carolina. "I'd been searching for low-fat stuff, and this really did the trick. I just always make sure I have them around."

Eating low-fat came relatively easy to Mikki, whose mother raised her on healthy fare. She never ate a lot of fried foods, always piled her plate with vegetables, and indulged in red meat only on occasion. So her cholesterol had always been healthy until 2 years ago, around the time she had a hysterectomy. Her cholesterol at that time hit a high of 213.

That her cholesterol was climbing at all made Mikki nervous. At the age of 12, she had open-heart surgery to open up her aorta. In 1993, she had a second surgery to replace two valves in her heart. "After all of that, I didn't want to have further problems because of cholesterol," Mikki says.

Mikki quickly doubled her efforts to eat better. She shopped for fat-free varieties of typically high-fat foods such as salad dressing. She gave up 2% milk in favor of the ½% variety and slathered her baked potatoes with Heinz 57 sauce instead of butter. She also made the difficult decision to give up chocolate, but she was happy to discover that foods like chocolate ice cream could be replaced with low-fat chocolate yogurt and that brownies and chocolate cakes could be made with low-fat ingredients.

But it was Tootsie Rolls that satisfied her spontaneous chocolate cravings. Now, instead of downing a small bag of M&M's, her previous chocolate of choice, she eats five or six little Tootsie Rolls—with no remorse. Her cholesterol now stands at 185. And since the Tootsie Rolls she buys are half the size of the ones she used to get, Mikki enjoys the luxury of knowing she can eat as many as 12 and get just 3 percent of her day's quota of saturated fat and no cholesterol. "I think that's a pretty good deal," she says.

W I N N I N G   A C T I O N

Satisfy chocolate cravings with low-fat alternatives. Too many chocolate goodies—candies, cakes, and brownies, for instance—are high in total fat, saturated fat, and cholesterol. Searching the supermarket for treats that are low in all those things is well worth the effort. In addition to Tootsie Rolls, look for fat-free and low-fat cookies, snack cakes, ice cream, and other candies. If you must have your favorite higher-fat candy, buy the mini size and take your time eating it so you savor the flavor and don't automatically reach for more when it's gone.

+++

SHE CHANGED HER GAME PLAN—AND WON

Once in a while, Nancy Vinson treats herself to chicken nuggets at a fast-food restaurant. But she'll never order a sandwich. She'd really rather not eat anything that comes on a bun.

Since 1998, Nancy, a 52-year-old Atlanta homemaker, has fought high cholesterol by closely monitoring her carbohydrate intake. Once a self-proclaimed "bread addict," she now limits herself to just two slices a day. She's equally cautious about other high-carbohydrate foods, including produce. She sticks with low-carb vegetables such as green beans, broccoli, brussels sprouts, cabbage, cauliflower, red and green peppers, and radishes. She limits herself to one piece of fruit per day. Instead of fruit juice, she drinks lots of water—seven 8-ounce glasses a day.

This sort of diet isn't for everyone. But it helped Nancy improve her cholesterol profile when more conventional dietary changes didn't seem to work.

Nancy learned she had high cholesterol in 1993. But she didn't take steps to control it until 1998, when her total cholesterol reached 247 and her triglycerides climbed to 210.

At her doctor's suggestion, Nancy tried following a low-fat diet. For 3 months, she limited her fat intake to 40 grams a day. To her surprise, and her doctor's, her total cholesterol rose to 252. "It was so frustrating," she recalls. "I thought I'd done the right thing diet-wise. I wondered, What's going on?"

Not wanting to see her cholesterol go higher, Nancy agreed to take Zocor. Within 3 months, her reading had dropped to 166, but at a price: She had severe leg cramps.

In the meantime, Nancy did some research into diet's impact on cholesterol. She discovered that in some people, a high carbohydrate intake can raise cholesterol. She asked her doctor to halve her daily dose of Zocor because of the side effects. Then she started a diet that restricted carbohydrates to 80 grams a day. Three months later, she had her cholesterol checked again. Her total cholesterol stood at 206, at bit higher than it had been, but very close to a healthy level. As Nancy notes, "It proved to me that if you're on the right diet, you don't need as much medication."

Nancy did try going off Zocor completely. When she relied on diet alone, her cholesterol bounced back to 230, where it remains to this day. She would like to get it to a healthier level, which is why she has added strength training to her aerobic exercise regimen. It must be helping: While her total cholesterol is holding steady, her LDL has dropped from a high of 177 to 163, and her HDL has risen from 36 to 49. Just as noteworthy, her triglycerides have plummeted to 91. A recent artery scan showed that she has minimal plaque buildup. And she's still off Zocor, although she says she'd take it again if her total cholesterol increased.

While she's proud of what she has accomplished, Nancy knows she has to continue working hard to control her cholesterol. And she takes that very seriously. Her mother died of an apparent heart attack at 42; her father also died young.

"I'm not going to let that happen to me," she says. "That's part of my motivation."

WINNING ACTION

Reevaluate your dietary changes as necessary. To control cholesterol, most experts recommend limiting fat, especially saturated fat. But it doesn't work for everyone. Some people, like Nancy, do better when they shift their attention to carbohydrates. That's because in some cases, a high carbohydrate intake can reduce HDL and elevate triglycerides. If you have high triglycerides, the American Heart Association recommends that you limit carbs to 50 percent of your total daily calories.

+++

SACRIFICING SUGAR KNOCKED HIS TRIGLYCERIDES COLD

Brian Ledoux, of Charlton, Massachusetts, is only 30 years old, but he's already found a strong incentive to keep his cholesterol and triglyceride levels under control. "My wife and I were having our first child, and I decided I wanted to be around as long as I could," he says.

He knew he had his work cut out for him, especially since his father's side of the family has a history of heart disease. As for Brian, back in 1997, his total cholesterol level was at 240, his HDL level was a mere 17, and his triglyceride reading was over 1,000. What's worse, Brian says that his cholesterol had been at those levels "for at least 3 years."

In many cases, elevated triglycerides are associated with low HDL. Brian's triglycerides were so high that his nutritionist suggested he do everything he could to knock them into line.

Since triglycerides can be elevated by the consumption of simple sugars and alcohol, Brian gave up alcohol completely. More important, he worked to remove refined sugars and white flour from his diet. "I stopped eating foods such as cookies and cakes," he says. "There are a lot of diabetic foods that I now eat." He also added flaxseed to his diet to help stabilize his blood sugar levels.

All this change was achieved without too much disruption for his wife and child. "My family has not really had to adjust too much as a result of my diet," says Brian. "We eat some different foods, but our main meals are the same."

By the end of 2000, Brian had made great progress toward great cholesterol health. His total cholesterol level was down to 150, and his triglyceride level was a fraction of the old at 190. (His HDL had inched up to 25, an improvement, but still on the low side.) By removing the sugars from his diet, he had also lost 25 pounds, bringing the weight on his 6-foot-1 frame down to 185.

Even when the numbers decline, he knows that he can't consider the battle won. Says Brian, "The biggest thing for me was to understand that this is a lifestyle change, not just a diet."

WINNING ACTION

Cut out refined sugars and grains. Simple sugars like those found in cookies, cakes, and hard candy give the body a quick energy burst—but sugars that go unused by the body are either stored as fat or converted into triglycerides by your liver. White flour causes similar problems since it is treated like a simple sugar by your body. Even if you don't eliminate sweets and refined-flour products, you can make them healthier for you. Start by using one-third less sugar than recipes call for, then cut back further if you like the results. For more fiber, replace half the white flour in pancakes, breads, and other baked goods with whole wheat. You'll barely notice the taste difference, but you'll reap significant cholesterol and triglyceride benefits.

++

SHE PARED POINTS
WITH PORTION CONTROL

Cozying up with a plate of cheese and crackers used to be a nightly ritual for Eileen Portz-Shovlin. Not anymore. She suspended her evening snacking in 1988, after her first cholesterol test yielded some unexpected results.

Despite being a long-distance runner who has logged about 40 miles a week for the past 21 years, Eileen had a total cholesterol level of 246, with an LDL reading of 163 and HDL of 70. "I was very surprised," says the 54-year-old magazine editor from Allentown, Pennsylvania. "I exercised a lot, and I thought I was a fairly good eater. I considered myself very healthy."

Upon examining her diet more closely, however, Eileen found some room for improvement. Cheese was among her weaknesses, as was butter. She used it liberally when cooking, and slathered it on baked potatoes and toast.

With a cholesterol level considered high, Eileen knew she had to cut back. Whenever possible, she substituted olive oil for butter when preparing meals, and topped her toast with jelly. She wasn't ready to give up cheese, but she abstained a couple of nights a week. She made other dietary changes, too, eating more fish, fruits, and vegetables, and less meat.

Even though Eileen had made significant improvements in her diet, her cholesterol wouldn't budge. Her doctor suggested that she take cholesterol-lowering medication, but she refused. "I believed that if I tried really hard, I could get my LDL down to a healthier level," she says.

Then in 1998, Eileen's mother underwent bypass surgery.

Her experience persuaded Eileen to become even more vigilant about her own eating habits. Not that she gave up all of her favorite foods. She just learned to be satisfied with less.

Cheese and crackers remains Eileen's favorite nighttime snack. Only now, she limits the cheese to no more than 2 ounces. "You can get pretty many slices if you make them really thin!" she says. Likewise, she allows herself just a sliver of butter for her baked potato, adding a little salt and pepper to enhance the flavor.

These changes have successfully nudged Eileen's cholesterol closer to healthier levels. While her total cholesterol remains above the 200 mark (219), her LDL has fallen to 126, and her HDL has held steady at 70.

Eileen would like to get her LDL below 120. But with a ratio (a comparison of total cholesterol to HDL) of 3.1, she's pleased with the progress she has made so far. What's more, she has no plans to give up her beloved cheese and butter for good. "I don't want to be too strict with my diet," she explains. "I need to treat myself on occasion. I can't deny myself the foods I love."

WINNING ACTION

Enjoy your favorite foods in sensible portions. Just because you're trying to lower your cholesterol doesn't mean you need to give up all your indulgences. In fact, a diet that seems like a series of dreary sacrifices is almost bound to fail. So don't be afraid to enjoy your treats of choice—be they cheese, chocolate, potato chips, or something else. Just keep the portion small, and chew slowly, so you can savor every delicious bite. That way, you'll feel satisfied with less.

+++

HE BROKE OFF
HIS LOVE AFFAIR WITH BURGERS

Mention Ty's Diner to Larry Barrett, and he'll tell you that it's "a great hangout with great burgers." From the smile on his face and the chuckle in his voice, you'll know that he has more than a passing familiarity with the place.

Ty's is something of a landmark in Larry's hometown of Wichita, Kansas. The restaurant's cheeseburgers and french fries won Larry's heart back in the late 1950s, when he was just a high school student and Ty's was *the* local hangout. Long after he graduated and established himself as an accountant, Larry and his high school buddies continued to go to Ty's for lunch.

Despite being a dedicated athlete (he recorded 16,000 miles in his running log, including 75 marathons since the 1970s), Larry had a diet that was nearly his undoing. "I would stop by Ty's once or twice a week for a cheeseburger, and if I got it to go, the grease would soak through the sack before I got out the door," he laughs. What's more, he kept his home freezer stocked with a side of beef, and he grilled steaks every weekend. He shouldn't have been surprised that by the early 1980s, his total cholesterol was approaching 260.

Despite a cholesterol level that put him at risk for a heart attack, Larry didn't make any changes to his diet. Instead, he stepped up the intensity of his running regimen. It helped, reducing his total cholesterol to 234.

Then in 1989, a friend and fellow runner invited Larry to join him for a week at a residential fitness center in Utah. Larry attended classes on nutrition and exercise, and was introduced to a diet free of animal protein. The experience persuaded him to reduce his meat consumption and to forgo his frequent trips to Ty's. "At first, I'd sit down to a salad, and I'd think, Boy, I'd sure like to have some meat with this," he says. "But eventually, it wasn't a big deal."

Even though Larry improved his eating habits, his heart was already in serious danger. In 1991, a cardiologist discovered that Larry's left descending artery was blocked. Larry underwent a procedure in which the artery-clogging plaque was sliced through with a diamond-tipped drill. The procedure had to be repeated twice more, the third time coupled with angioplasty to reduce scarring. After that, Larry began taking Lipitor. His total cholesterol quickly dropped to 190 and, over the next few years, would inch even lower.

In 1994, with his doctor's approval, Larry stopped taking Lipitor. He wanted to try controlling his cholesterol through diet and exercise. His total cholesterol climbed slightly, from 151 to 163. And it stayed there.

Certainly, Larry's exercise program deserves some of the credit. He continued his running regimen until 2000, when hip pain forced him to stop. In its place, he took up bicycling and lap swimming.

But since he's always led an active lifestyle, Larry—who's now 63—is convinced that his healthier diet has made a big difference. "I eat mostly chicken and fish, fresh vegetables, beans, and rice," he says proudly. "I seldom have red meat—and I don't miss it, either."

That's not to say that Larry has totally forsaken his former haunt. He admits to stopping by Ty's for a cheeseburger and onion rings. But his visits come three or four times a year, not once or twice a week. "When I go, it's a special occasion," he smiles. "And I really enjoy it."

WINNING ACTION

Reserve your favorite restaurant meal as a special treat. Eating out used to be a big deal. These days, it's routine, because it fits so well into the modern on-the-go lifestyle. But if your tastes run to high-fat, high-cholesterol fare, as

Larry's did, you may be harming your heart for the sake of convenience. No matter what your choice of restaurants, scan the menu for items labeled as "heart smart" or "low-fat." And watch your portion sizes: A proper portion may be one-half to one-quarter of the entrée that's served. Save the less nutritious fare for special occasions—and then savor every bite!

+++

HE STOPPED DIETING
AND LOST THE WEIGHT

Twenty years ago, Robert Wilson lost 100 pounds, largely by eating a lot of salad. Nineteen years ago, he gained back all 100 pounds.

"I don't like salads anymore," he admits. "I lost weight by eating stuff I don't like. It wasn't a diet I would stay on."

Robert, a 70-year-old West Hills, California, resident, may not eat salads. But those 100 pounds are gone—forever, he says. At 6 feet 4 inches, he weighs 253, down from a high of 360. And in the bargain, his cholesterol, which had never been high, dropped nearly 30 points, from 158 in November 1995 to 132 in February 2001. His HDL went from 33 to 39; his LDL, once 95, is down to 67. And his triglycerides, unacceptable at 186 in November 1995, are 134.

Robert watches what he eats. Cheese spread, which he used to eat by the jarful, is out, as are steaks and beer. After-dinner treats such as cookies and cakes are all low-fat.

But he does not force himself to consume foods that don't please his palate. "I enjoy what I eat," he says. "I tried to eat a lot of salad, and now I wouldn't touch it."

Instead, Robert enjoys low-fat frozen dinners several nights a week. "A lot of people ask me how I can stand them, but I find them quite tasty," he says. He has several servings of fruit a day and, to satisfy those cheese cravings, eats low-fat cottage cheese. He also drinks a lot of water.

Robert, a retired aerospace project engineer, started gaining weight in his forties. After hitting a high of 360 in 1995, he tried to slim down, once again working salads into his meals and pedaling an exercise bike. But that fall, after finding out that he had two blocked arteries, he began to diet and exercise in earnest.

After undergoing angioplasty in April 1996, he used a treadmill and weight room as part of his rehabilitation. Today, he visits the gym every Monday, Wednesday, and Friday, spending 20 minutes on the treadmill and 40 minutes in the weight room, lifting free weights and operating several weight-lifting machines. "My stomach is as hard as a rock, and I have muscles where there weren't muscles before," he says.

In addition, he says, he feels great. Regular checkups with the cardiologist are always good, and annual stress tests show no more blockages.

And best of all, the heartburn that was a regular nuisance is gone. "You know how people who smoke won't go outside without their cigarettes?" Robert says. "I was like that with Rolaids. I never went out without a roll. I don't even carry Rolaids anymore."

WINNING ACTION

Don't force yourself to eat foods you don't like. Nothing is more discouraging than sitting down to a long-anticipated meal and realizing that there is nothing on the table to tickle your tastebuds. Fruits and vegetables come in endless variety; if you don't like one, try another. And there are ways to enhance dishes that might not initially entice you. If regular salads leave you cold, for example, liven them up with pickled beets, sunflower seeds, grapefruit and orange sections, tangy vinegars, cooked

*beans, or herbs. Edible flowers such as violets and nastur-
tiums add flavor as well as eye appeal, which shouldn't be
underestimated as an appetite enhancer.*

++

HIS EATING HABITS ARE
HIS CONSTANT COMPANION

Wherever Gene Solyntjes ventures, he never forgets his
healthy eating habits. They're with him whether he's working
hard in his office, ordering a meal in a restaurant, or flying
across the country. They've helped him shave 64 points from
his cholesterol—and 43 pounds from his 5-foot-9 frame.

As an orthotist (he designs ands fits orthotic devices and
braces), Gene often tells his clients to slim down. But he
never heeded his own advice. When he had a mild heart attack in March 2000, he weighed 232 pounds. "I imagined I'd
end up like my father, who died of a heart attack when he was
only 52," he says.

As soon as he was able, Gene enrolled in a special program
at the health club he belongs to in Seattle, where he lives.
Called 20/20, the 12-week program helps clients improve
their health through nutrition, exercise, and weight loss.

Gene's primary goal was to take off his extra pounds. But
he also hoped to improve his cholesterol profile. At the time,
his total cholesterol was 227, with an LDL level of 153 and
an HDL level of 48. His triglycerides measured 130. The
numbers weren't all that bad, but to someone who had already suffered one heart attack, they were ripe for improvement.

Once in the program, Gene began exercising 5 to 7 days a
week, either at the health club or at home on his treadmill.
And his diet received a major makeover. "Before my heart
attack, my eating habits were awful," he admits. "I'd starve
myself during the day because I thought I was just too busy

to stop for a meal. Then I'd chow down big at night. I'd say my eating habits have changed 95 percent."

On his new diet, Gene builds his meals around fresh fruits and vegetables, as well as lean meats. He makes an effort to consume between 30 and 40 percent of his total calories before 10 o'clock each morning, so he has the energy to get through the day. He pays close attention to his fat and carbohydrate intakes, too.

Because he's often on the go, Gene has developed special strategies to keep his eating habits on track in any situation. Each morning, he whips up a blender drink of fruit (whatever he has around), olive oil, water, and sometimes peanut butter or cottage cheese for protein. He pours the concoction into an insulated container and takes it to work, where he drinks it before 10:00 A.M. He also carries his lunch from home: a salad of deeply colored greens, sprinkled with olive oil and balsamic vinegar.

On those occasions when he eats out, Gene looks for lean meat entrées. If he gets a salad, he requests the dressing on the side. And he always passes on dessert. "Dessert is great—for other people," he laughs.

Even when he travels, Gene remains vigilant about his eating habits. "If I'm flying somewhere, I request low-fat meals when I reserve my tickets," he says.

Gene's perseverance has been rewarded with a cholesterol profile that anyone would be proud of. His total cholesterol has stabilized at 163, with an LDL of 103 and an HDL of 47. His triglycerides have sunk to 63. And he's taken off the pounds he wanted to: At age 58, he's a trim 189 pounds.

WINNING ACTION

Wherever you go, take your diet with you. Don't let a trip away from home distance you from your cholesterol-conscious eating habits. Many restaurants and airlines of-

fer low-fat meals; some have specially designed light menus on hand for the asking. When such options aren't available, lighten up your meal by steering clear of fried foods, fatty meats, heavy salad dressings, and desserts.

+++

SHAPE UP YOUR
CHOLESTEROL PROFILE

✦ ✦ ✦

HE TOOK ONE STEP AT A TIME—
AND NOW HE COVERS MILES

As a bookkeeper at a New York City stock firm, Mike Cesare lived under a lot of stress: 14-hour workdays, eating on the run, daily subway commutes from Copiague on Long Island into Manhattan. He retired in 1989, but by then, he says, "the damage had already been done."

By 1992, Mike was living with constant chest pain. "It got to the point where I literally couldn't walk five steps without pain," he says. "I was popping nitros [nitroglycerin tablets] like they were peanuts."

Plagued by high blood pressure and a total cholesterol level over 300, he underwent triple bypass surgery that year. It was as if a new world opened for him. "It was like a second chance," says Mike. "You can't believe that you don't have pain anymore." And he was determined never to cause such damage to himself again.

A week and a half after getting home from the hospital, he

decided that to keep his heart in good shape he would start walking. At first, it was an effort just to reach the end of his block and return. But even though that was a modest endeavor, he kept at it.

Within a few months, Mike was making trips to and from a supermarket a mile away. And he discovered that his body was not just tolerating the exercise, it was thriving on it. "My body said to me, like in that Peggy Lee song, 'Is that all there is?'" he says. "My body wasn't satisfied with the 2 miles and wanted more."

After getting encouragement from a jogger he regularly passed, Mike added a bit of running to his routine and began participating in half-marathons (13.1-mile races). After years of walking experience, this 72-year-old now covers 40 miles a week, walking 8 to 10 miles per day. As a result, his total cholesterol is under 200, and his weight has dropped from 235 pounds to 195.

What's more, he also participates in four bowling leagues and regularly works as the announcer for local high school football and basketball games.

"Don't expect immediate results," says Mike. "Even if you lose only 1 pound every 2 or 3 weeks, that's still 20 pounds a year. It makes a difference. It adds up."

WINNING ACTION

Start slowly and build up. If you're recovering from heart disease or overcoming years of physical inactivity, your body won't have much endurance. Pushing yourself too hard at the beginning might cause you to pull muscles, lose your breath—or worse. Have patience with your body's limitations. Before you know it, you'll have the strength to walk, swim, run, and bike beyond your wildest dreams.

++

DON'T JUST LIE THERE—MOVE!

In the old days, Ernest Laabs finished off a good meal by plopping down on the couch in front of the television. These days, he's more apt to take a 15-minute walk after every one of his meals. "The object is to get the body moving and circulating, just to get all this stuff moving," says the 69-year-old San Bernardino, California, resident.

Ernest had a massive heart attack in 1991, and his cholesterol hit 350. "The doctors told me that if I behaved, I could live maybe another 5 years," Ernest recalls. Five years later, he was diagnosed with diabetes.

By the summer of 2000, Ernest was taking 27 pills a day to control his myriad ailments, which by then included high blood pressure. He also had a calcified artery in his leg, which kept him up nights, pacing in pain. An outspoken friend of his wife, Elayne, took a look at him one day and asked her if she was prepared to spend the rest of her life alone. That was all Elayne needed to drag her husband to the NewStart Lifestyle Program in Weimar, California, a facility that helps patients improve their health through diet and exercise. "I was not pleased with the idea of going," Ernest says. "I said, 'This has got to be a joke.' But I went because I promised I'd love, honor, and obey her."

After 18 days at the NewStart program, Ernest returned home a changed person. He eliminated steak, his favorite food, from his diet altogether. He also gave up cheese, eggs, and butter, and switched from regular milk to soy milk. Now he builds his meals around tofu, homemade grain breads, and fresh fruits and vegetables.

He also learned to take a 15-minute walk after every meal. Sometimes, he simply paces his 2,000-square-foot house or goes up and down the stairs. Other times, he walks around the yard or circles the neighborhood. "You don't need a park to walk," Ernest says. "You just have to get out there and do it."

Improvements in his diet and exercise have made it easier

for Ernest to enjoy his favorite activity: square dancing. "It used to tucker me out like you wouldn't believe," he says. "If I danced straight for 15 minutes, it was great. Now, I could dance all evening. On New Year's Eve, I danced from 7:30 to 12:30. I didn't want to quit, but everybody else did."

He also cut down the pills he takes to just three a day—none of which are for his cholesterol, which dropped most recently to 155. His leg no longer bothers him at all, and he shed 16 pounds in the 6 months after he went to Weimar. At 5 feet 10 inches, he now weighs 164 pounds.

WINNING ACTION

Take a short walk after every meal. Rather than slump in front of the TV after eating, commit yourself to doing some activity, be it a short walk in the house or a longer one outdoors. By moving immediately after eating, you'll sneak in some extra exercise. And for those with diabetes, the exercise helps stabilize blood sugars after eating. If lying on the couch is your habit, ask your spouse or a friend to encourage you, even join you. Ask someone else to hide the remote control. Get dressed for your walk before dinner or paste a big reminder note on the refrigerator. The goal is to create a new habit of exercise.

++

AN EXERCISE JOURNAL TELLS HIM HOW HE'S DOING

When Bill Grant finishes a bike ride, he pulls out a raggedy spiral notebook and records the date, the miles he rode, and the speed he did it in. Keeping an exercise log helps Bill track his progress and gives him something to strive toward every week, month, and year.

Bill took up biking in 1995 after a car accident forced him to get hip replacement surgery. Bill had to give up the activities he loved most, which included racquetball and jogging. A life without competitive sports seemed unthinkable to this former college football player. "If you've ever played sports, that competitive feeling never goes away," says Bill, 48, who is president of the Hildebrandt Learning Centers in Dallas, Pennsylvania.

His doctor suggested biking or swimming instead, and Bill chose biking. About a year after he started riding, he bought an odometer. "I would keep track of the time and my average speed and try to compare it each time," he says. "But after a while, I couldn't keep track of it in my mind, so I started keeping it in a book." With help from his exercise log, Bill found a new competitor: himself.

In 1998, just 4 minutes into his ride on a stationary bike at the gym, Bill started having chest pains. At first, he attributed it to his chest cold. But the pain spread to his shoulders and down his left arm. "It was like somebody was grabbing the middle of my chest," he recalls.

Bill learned that one of his arteries was 95 percent blocked and had a stent implanted to keep it propped open. A few other arteries were also showing signs of blockage, and Bill's cholesterol was at an all-time high of 254. Once again, Bill's competitive nature kicked in, and he became determined to lower his cholesterol. "The doctor said he was going to hook me up with a handicapped license plate," he says. "And other people were saying, 'Oh, you won't be able to do much; you'll have to relax.' And I said, 'There's no way I'm going to do that.' There was no way I was going to let my cholesterol stay high."

Bill began exercising 5 days a week. In addition to biking, he took up weight lifting. He also made some dietary changes. He gave up chocolate, red meat, and butter, and switched from 2% milk to fat-free milk. He ate more whole wheat breads, whole grain cereals, and fish, turkey, and chicken. He also took a tablespoon of milled flaxseed every day.

Over the course of 7 months, with a little help from Lipitor, Bill saw his cholesterol drop to 154. It still hovers there, give or take a few points.

These days, he logs at least 70 to 90 miles a week on his bike, increasing to 100 to 120 miles in the summer months. In 2000, he rode a total of 1,500 miles, a feat that he'd like to repeat. "I'm always trying to better my mileage," he says. "It's just my competitive nature. I always want to see if I can do better."

WINNING ACTION

Keep track of your exercise in a log. Whether you write down the minutes you ride, the distance you run, or the amount of weight you lift, an exercise journal helps you realize how far you've come and provides a measuring stick for goals. It's also a great way to create some competition with your own accomplishments.

++

SHE FOUND A PARTNER
WHO KEEPS HER ON HER TOES

In the early 1990s, Lita Batistoni was regularly donating blood for her mother, who had non-Hodgkin's lymphoma. This meant Lita's cholesterol was being checked regularly. By all accounts, she had no cause for concern. Even though her father and brother had high cholesterol, Lita's reading hovered comfortably between the high 160s and low 170s.

By January 2000, though, her family history had caught up with her. During a routine physical, she learned that her total cholesterol had climbed to 250, with an LDL level of 174 and a ratio (a comparison of total cholesterol to HDL) of 4.9:1. "I ate fairly healthfully, though I loved snacks and sweets. And I wasn't exercising that much," says 53-year-old Lita, who lives in Hampton, New Jersey. "When I learned I had high cholesterol, I realized it could be a real problem as I got older. And I wanted to stay healthy for my family."

She started reading nutrition labels and cutting out the sweet, high-saturated-fat snacks that she loved. And she tried to get into the swing of exercising, engaging in moderate walking and using a treadmill on and off during the first half of 2000.

But Lita's biggest success came through a Jazzercise course that she didn't even want to sign up for. "My 17-year-old daughter, Holly, was the one who was interested in it, and she motivated me to go ahead and try it," she says.

After one class, Lita was hooked, not just because the class was invigorating but also because she loved the company around her. "I thought it was a good form of exercise because we were doing this with other women," she says. "It wasn't like just going out to take a walk by yourself. I felt the group effort was more of what I needed to motivate me."

The other exercisers may inspire Lita, but her daughter remains her biggest exercise influence. After working 10 hours, Lita will come home ready for nothing more than a good nap, but that's not to be. "My daughter will be changed and prodding me to go," she says. "And after doing an hour of high-impact aerobics, I'll feel so good that I've gone."

By June 2000, Lita's total cholesterol reading was down to 204, and her LDL level had dropped by almost a third to 128. Her doctor felt good enough about the improvement to wait another year before checking her again.

Her doctor isn't the only one giving her compliments. Lita's son, Russell, who lifts weights for a U.S. Marine–sponsored program offered at his high school, tells her she looks much better since she began exercising. "My husband, Frank, says I look more toned, too," says Lita. "And now I've convinced him to walk with me on my days off." It's amazing what partners will do for you.

WINNING ACTION

Find an exercise partner. With a spouse, sibling, friend, or neighbor exercising at your side, you're more likely to stick to a program and achieve long-term success. The two of you will spur each other on, give encouragement when necessary, and, perhaps most important, have someone to talk to so that your exercise time passes more quickly.

++

HE HIRED A TRAINER
TO HELP HIM STAY ON TRACK

In the summer of 1999, Craig Weintraub found the help he needed to whip himself into shape and knock his cholesterol down to manageable levels.

"As I was getting older, I was doing less physical activity, and at 163 pounds, I was probably the heaviest I had ever been," says Craig, a 45-year-old Palmer, Pennsylvania, resident. "Even after 8 hours of sleep, I was still tired." Since his mother had passed away of heart disease, his father had had a stroke, and his own LDL cholesterol level had hit 171, he knew that he needed to change his ways.

"I wanted to lose weight and get in shape to both look and feel better," says Craig. "And if I was going to feel better, I could only do it two ways: eating better and exercising."

In terms of diet, he dropped fast food and high-saturated-fat snacks and started making meals with beans, chicken, and organic rice and other grains. "I realized that cooking didn't take up as much time as I thought it did," he says.

The exercise had an even greater impact than the diet,

thanks to the efforts of one Yonny Acevedo, a personal trainer at Formula Fitness in nearby Easton. "If it weren't for him, I don't think I would have achieved the results that I did," says Craig. "It's one thing to go to the gym at 6:30, 7:00 in the morning and another thing to go there and have a personal trainer push your butt for an hour."

Craig had already used free weights at home to shed some extra pounds, and that spurred his desire to do more. By hiring Yonny, he says, "I knew that I would have someone to help me to use the equipment correctly and to give me that push."

By summer 2000, Craig had dropped 33 pounds from his 5-foot-9 frame (and gained 20 pounds of muscle). He also lowered his LDL cholesterol to 101. "People are amazed at the physical change that occurred in less than a year," he says. "I went to the tailor, and he said, 'You're the only one I've seen that's brought his suits in to have them taken in.'"

In addition to increasing his physical strength, Craig says that he now feels rested after 6 hours of sleep, and he doesn't worry about occasionally breaking from his diet. "If I go out to a nice restaurant and want a dessert, I'll order it," he says, "because I know I'm going to be at the gym the next day."

WINNING ACTION

Hire a personal trainer. Many gyms offer lists of qualified trainers, but before you sign up with one, ask for references from other individuals whom he or she has helped. Ask these people how the trainer worked with them, accepted setbacks, and changed the program over time. In addition to teaching you how to maximize your workouts on exercise machines and in the weight room, trainers give you someone else to answer to. They push you to take better care of yourself and provide positive reassurance with each step you take—all of which encourages you to do more!

++

SHE PUTS WALKING FIRST—
BY DOING IT FIRST THING

When Bonnie Luft says that walking is a priority, she means it. First thing in the morning, she downs a glass of orange juice and heads out for a 4-mile walk. "I just throw on my clothes and step out the door," says the 52-year-old resident of Waco, Texas.

High cholesterol caught Bonnie by surprise in 1999, when a routine blood test found that her cholesterol level had soared to 340, the highest it had ever been. It had hovered around 240 for the previous 3 years, but she never did anything about it. "My doctor said, 'I know you're okay, you're eating right, and you're exercising,'" she recalls. "So I wasn't all that concerned."

Bonnie had always taken care of her health. As a senior lecturer on health, human performance, and recreation at Baylor University, she taught dance aerobics at least twice a week, as she'd done for 25 years, and walked a couple of miles three or four times a week. She ate a healthy diet, avoiding high-fat foods such as desserts and eating chicken or fish instead of red meat. But 340 was a scary number, and she was at a loss as to what else she could do. "Here I was in health and fitness, and I had high cholesterol," she says.

Bonnie started taking the drug Lipitor and a daily aspirin. She also began taking longer, more frequent walks, increasing her distance from 2 miles to 4. Every morning, during the months when she isn't teaching, she walks about an hour. During the school year, she strives to go at least three times a week. Only a life-changing event like her daughter's wedding in January 2001 managed to keep Bonnie from her regular walks. "It stays on the top of my priority list," she says. "When I don't walk, I miss it."

Most days, she walks along a nature trail near her house. On days when the weather is bad, she walks on an indoor track at the campus or heads to a nearby mall. And on those

rare occasions when she just can't get out in the morning, she
goes in the evening instead.

Bonnie's determination has worked. Two months after her
cholesterol hit 340, it dropped down to 190, and these days, it
hovers around 205. Keeping it down, however, doesn't come
easily even for someone as active as Bonnie. "I really have to
work at it," she says. "I have to eat right, and I have to walk."

WINNING ACTION

*Walk before doing anything else. Take your walks first thing
in the morning, when your schedule is most clear. You'll be
less apt to cancel in favor of something else if you walk
first. So if something tempting does come up, you will already have done your exercise for the day.*

++

CHOLESTEROL IS NO MATCH
FOR HER MUSCLE

When Jennifer Reisinger learned she had high cholesterol,
she turned to exercise—specifically, strength training—to get
it under control. Her therapy of choice came as no surprise to
those who knew her. After all, daily workouts helped Jennifer
overcome a 2-year battle with agoraphobia, a paralyzing fear
of the outside world.

Between 1990 and 1992, Jennifer seldom left her Sheboy-
gan, Wisconsin, apartment, whiling away the hours by watching TV. Finally, her parents convinced her to see a therapist,
who suggested exercise to help her anxiety. "My parents
bought me a step bench and aerobics videos," she recalls.
"Soon, my day wasn't complete unless I did my workout."
She enjoyed being active, and she felt better about herself.
Eventually, she was able to venture outside without fear.

By the end of 1992, with her agoraphobia under control, Jennifer faced a new challenge: high cholesterol. "I was only in my early thirties, so I was a little surprised," she recalls. "I didn't worry about it, though. I just continued my daily workouts, and I tried to cut back on fat."

Over the next 2 years, Jennifer's cholesterol stayed in the neighborhood of 230, with an HDL level between 54 and 64, LDL between 151 and 167, and triglycerides around 100. By 1994, she had cut out all fried foods, and she had begun using hand weights in her aerobic workouts. Even with these changes, her cholesterol dropped just 3 points in 3 years.

"My doctor kept telling me to either get it under 200 or see a dietitian," Jennifer says. "I didn't want professional help, and I didn't want medication. But I was getting so frustrated."

Through her own research, she learned that high cholesterol may be associated with intramuscular fat, which is best lost through strength training. In 1998, deciding that she had nothing to lose, she invested in a workout station with barbells, plus a set of dumbbells. Twice a week, she replaced her usual aerobics session with a 1-hour, full-body strength-training session.

Jennifer got the results she wanted. By 1999, her total cholesterol had sunk to 190. "I was so thrilled that I bought heavier weights and increased the length of my strength-training sessions," she says. According to her most recent test, her total cholesterol has dropped 18 more points, to 172. Her HDL stands at 77, and her LDL has fallen to 83. Likewise, her triglycerides have plummeted from a high of 117 all the way to 58.

"When I got that last test result, I was so happy I cried," Jennifer says. "You just think you're never going to get there." She felt so inspired by her personal success that she has earned her certification as a nutrition and fitness consultant. At age 42, she has taken her consulting online and is poised to show others how they can win the cholesterol war, too.

W I N N I N G   A C T I O N

Pick up some weights to outmuscle cholesterol. Many people avoid strength training for fear that they'll end up looking like Arnold Schwarzenegger. Lifting a modest amount of weight won't create bulk, but it will build muscle. That can help improve your cholesterol profile and shed pounds. After all, the more muscle you have, the more calories you burn. And according to the National Heart, Lung, and Blood Institute, doing any physical activity for even a few minutes a day can make your HDL rise and your LDL fall. If you're new to strength training, your best bet is to consult a personal trainer to learn proper technique. Your doctor may be able to recommend a qualified professional; if not, check at a health club or YMCA.

++

HIS TRAVEL PLANS SENT CHOLESTEROL PACKING

Joe Miranda's idea of a vacation is a 7-day bicycle tour of the Rocky Mountains. While pedaling a bike for 60 to 80 miles a day may not seem all that relaxing, Joe can't think of a better way to spend his time off.

Active vacations have become an annual event for Joe and his wife. They browse brochures and search Web sites until they find a bicycle tour that appeals to them. Then they start their training.

For Joe, a 60-year-old retired computer specialist, the tours are an opportunity to indulge his sense of adventure. They also add purpose to his workouts. "As much as I enjoy exercising, if it doesn't have a goal, I end up asking myself, Why am I doing this?" he says.

In fact, Joe has a very good reason to keep himself fit. In

1994, he underwent an emergency quadruple bypass. After the surgery, he learned that his cholesterol profile was seriously out of whack. At 160, his total cholesterol seemed perfectly healthy. But his LDL of 130 was borderline high, while his HDL of 20 was much too low. "I knew these numbers had to change," he says. "I certainly didn't want another bypass—or worse yet, a heart attack."

Even before the surgery, Joe had been cycling and running regularly. Post-bypass, he redoubled his efforts to stay fit. Twice a week, he'd hop on his bike for hour-long excursions around his St. Simons Island, Georgia, home. On alternate days, he'd run.

To this day, Joe follows the same exercise program. It's ambitious, to be sure. But Joe's motivation seldom falters, because he knows he's got to be ready for his next bicycle tour. Most recently, he and his wife took that 500-mile trip through the Rockies. "We worked our way up to it by going on less grueling excursions—weekend tours and 1-day rides—over the course of the year," Joe says. "We're always looking to sign up for shorter events as training."

Joe and his wife have also participated in the Bicycle Ride Across Georgia, with a route that stretches from Hartwell—a town northeast of Atlanta—to the coast south of Savannah. "Eventually, I want to sign up for a 100-mile 1-day ride in Maryland," Joe says.

Events like these have encouraged Joe to stick with his exercise regimen, which in turn has helped improve his cholesterol profile. As of 1999, his LDL dropped to 120, while his HDL rose to 35. He has maintained these numbers ever since, a feat that he attributes to a combination of regular vigorous physical activity, a low-fat diet, and medication (Lipitor).

Joe is keenly aware that bypass surgery likely saved his life. That's why he so relishes the opportunity to see the country from the seat of his bicycle—and to stay in shape while doing it. "I got a second chance," he says. "The rest is up to me."

W I N N I N G   A C T I O N

Don't take your vacation sitting down. Many tour companies offer walking and cycling packages to travelers who prefer more active itineraries. Often, individual tours are tailored to specific fitness levels, so you can select one that matches your skills and interests. Once you sign up, you can turn your fitness routine into a training regimen. You have a very specific goal to work toward, and that can be a powerful incentive for exercising regularly. By the time you're ready to depart for your destination of choice, your cholesterol just might be several points lower!

++

AS OIL PRICES RISE, HIS CHOLESTEROL PLUMMETS

In 1998, Bob Anderson and his wife decided to change their home's heating system from oil to wood. At the time, making the switch seemed like a good way to save money. Bob never imagined that it might also save his life.

Back then, Bob had just learned that his total cholesterol had climbed to a very risky 285. A trim 5 feet 5 inches and 152 pounds, he hardly looked like a candidate for heart disease. But he took his cholesterol reading very seriously.

"My doctor gave me a prescription for Lipitor—10 milligrams a day—along with the usual advice to eat better and exercise more," recalls the 34-year-old book assembly team manager from Hellertown, Pennsylvania. "I cleaned up my diet right away. I bought salads instead of fast food for lunch, and I gave up butter and late-night cheese steaks."

While these changes took effort, they never fazed Bob. He was more concerned about finding time to work out, especially with a family to care for. "I have three young daughters, so I can't easily fit an exercise program into my schedule," he explains. "I can't just take off bicycling or skiing." Even going to his company's on-site gym isn't an option. "If I spend an hour there, that's an hour less with my family," he says.

But when you live in an old farmhouse with a never-ending maintenance list, as Bob does, getting enough physical activity can be easier than expected. That was especially true once the Andersons started using wood heat, and Bob was collecting the wood himself.

"There's some family-owned property close to our home, with lots of trees," Bob says. "My brother-in-law and I would chop down the trees, saw them into logs, split the logs, and stack the wood." Since the Andersons go through lots of wood during cold Pennsylvania winters, keeping enough on hand is a year-round job. And Bob can do most of the work with his wife and children nearby.

Chopping wood isn't the only activity that helps keep Bob fit. He no longer trims the lawn with a riding mower, opting for a push mower instead. And he and his wife take their daughters for long walks around their hilly neighborhood about three times a week during the summer months.

Because of Bob's decidedly unconventional approach to fitness, he never had to sacrifice treasured family time for workout time. Over the course of a year, his total cholesterol dropped to 162. "Because I never had trouble with my weight, I didn't see any reason to go out of my way to exercise," he says. "Incorporating physical activity into my daily routine, and making that activity productive, seems to keep me on track."

Because he has a family history of high cholesterol, Bob continues to take Lipitor on his doctor's advice. He's proud that his cholesterol has held steady, as he deserves to be. "When you find out that your cholesterol is sky-high and you tell yourself, I need to do something, and a year later it's where it should be . . . there's real satisfaction in that," he says.

WINNING ACTION

*Put more oomph into your household chores. Many peo-
ple avoid exercising because they think they don't have
the time for it. But you don't need to spend an hour at the
local gym to get a good workout. Consider your daily routine: You're probably doing all sorts of activities that, with a
little extra vigor, can get your heart pumping and those
calories burning. For example, in one hour of activity, a
150-pound person can burn 204 calories walking the dog,
or 238 calories vacuuming the carpets, or 292 calories rak-
ing leaves. You'll pare points from your cholesterol and
pounds from your body just taking care of chores that
need to be done anyway!*

+++

SHE ADDED A LITTLE
AND GOT A LOT

Rebecca Sanders had her exercise regimen down pat: 30 minutes four times a week on either the treadmill or the recumbent bicycle. But her cholesterol level still was not what she
wanted. So she added an extra 10 minutes to her workouts.

"That 10 minutes really makes a difference," says Rebecca, a 50-year-old high school science teacher in Springfield, Ohio. "But you've got to be clipping along, working up
a sweat."

A few years ago, Rebecca's total cholesterol stood at 248.
Her doctor recommended nothing more than minor dietary
changes and a few aerobic workouts weekly.

Rebecca, however, was concerned. Her maternal grandfather, a biochemist, died of a heart attack in his early forties.
Her father, a physician, was always giving her literature and
tapes dealing with health matters. She knew she had to do
something different. Not only was her total cholesterol

higher than it should have been, but her chronic digestive problems were getting worse.

In 1999, Rebecca started experiencing severe pain in her stomach. Her doctors gave her pills for relief, but they made her very tired. Then, in the summer of 1999, she had several precancerous polyps removed from her upper colon. "That was the last straw," she says. "I finally decided I had to do something about my diet."

Many changes, such as adding acidophilus, a type of bacteria that supports digestion, and balancing carbohydrates and proteins, were intended to help her intestinal problems. "But it seems to me that treatments like these can have multiple benefits," she says. "What's good for one body system is good for them all."

Oatmeal is one food that has many benefits, including the ability to lower cholesterol. Rebecca has some for breakfast every morning. She also takes 1,000 milligrams of flaxseed oil every day. She cut out the peanuts she used to snack on, substituting almonds and pretzels. And when she feels compelled to eat a chocolate chip cookie, she selects one with oatmeal in it.

Of course, exercise has also played an important role in Rebecca's cholesterol management plan. She says that the most difficult part of her fitness routine is finding the time to do it. She sets aside 40 minutes in the morning to work out on the treadmill or bike. In the summer, she switches to swimming—1 mile about four times a week. She uses exercise machines about two or three times a week all year round. Rebecca adds that the workouts were easier after her doctor prescribed vitamins. "I was able to kick more butt," she says.

And she finds motivation for exercise in reflecting on how good she feels. "If I do what works for me, all my systems feel better," she says. "Then if I cheat, my body lets me know about it. I feel sluggish and irritable. For example, if I eat a hamburger, it is much harder for me to do the treadmill."

Rebecca's commitment to exercising regularly, and to eating well, shows in her cholesterol reading. Her total cholesterol is down to 201. Her advice to others: "When you are tempted to eat something you shouldn't, think, How many more miles will I have to do on the treadmill? Then you realize that it's not worth it."

WINNING ACTION

Add just 10 minutes to your workout. According to the American Medical Association, the more physical activity patients engage in, the greater the benefit they achieve. And introducing extra exercise in small increments may make maintaining a regular workout schedule easier. Aerobic exercise raises levels of HDL cholesterol and may reduce levels of LDL if accompanied by weight loss. Exercise also has other heart benefits: It strengthens the heart muscle, promotes weight loss, lowers blood pressure, and can also help reduce stress.

++

HE'S HALF THE MAN HE USED TO BE—AND LOVES IT!

A few years ago, Howard Riel was every doctor's nightmare. He weighed 430 pounds, smoked three to four packs of cigarettes a day, never thought about exercise, and sported a total cholesterol reading of 286. "I just figured I was tough and could be fat and smoke, and when I was 80, I would slow down, maybe lose a little weight," says Howard, a resident of St. Petersburg, Florida.

He barely made it to 40 before his unhealthy habits caught up with him. In March 1996, he had a heart attack. Once he was in the hospital, doctors found that several arteries were 90 percent blocked. They suggested a quadruple bypass, he says, "but I knew that if I had the surgery, I would die on the table."

Howard wheedled a 5-month reprieve out of the surgeon, during which he'd have to lose 100 pounds. He started immediately, walking around the nurses' station while hooked to a heart monitor. "The nurses checked my monitor and let me know whether I could keep walking or whether my heart needed to rest," he says.

In addition to cutting out smoking and adopting the Pritikin lifestyle program—a low-fat, high-fiber plan loaded with fruit, vegetables, and whole grains—Howard upped his activity level by meeting with a personal trainer and designing an exercise program.

Three weeks after leaving the hospital, Howard ached to do more than walk a treadmill and diet. Since he was still over 400 pounds and had to avoid high-impact exercises, he found an old bicycle and took to the streets. "I rode it every day and got the bug!" he says.

Within 6 months, Howard lost the 100 pounds and was able to avoid the bypass surgery. But he didn't stop there. On a picnic with his wife, he saw the annual Assault on Mt. Mitchell, a 102-mile bike endurance ride that ends with a climb of 11,000 feet up the mountain. "The cyclists would stop and fall on the ground in total exhaustion!" he says. "I need goals, and I decided right then and there to join them next year."

Howard and his wife have now completed the Assault three times. They have also run their first marathon at Disney World, and are planning to make it an annual event. Howard is already preparing for his next goal: the Paris-Brest-Paris, a 1,200-kilometer bike ride next held in 2003. "It's held every 4 years and is one of the largest amateur rides in the world," he says.

Ever since losing the weight, Howard has had no problem keeping himself at 200 pounds and his total cholesterol below 120. "People always ask me how I did it," he says. "I tell them, it's your choice. You choose either a banana or a hamburger. It's up to you."

WINNING ACTION

Pick up a bike and take to the road. Walking may be the activity most people think of when it comes to exercise, but biking can take you farther and to more exciting places. The distance you cover each day lets you explore new territory rather than merely circling the same blocks again and again. Biking is also easier on the joints than jogging or walking, so it's a great choice for overweight people who need to avoid putting pressure on their knees or hips. If you haven't been on a bike since elementary school, strap on a helmet and hit the road!

++

HE HIT THE ROAD AND LEFT HIS CHOLESTEROL IN THE DUST

In December 1999, after learning his cholesterol was 264 and his blood pressure was slightly elevated, Nacho Perez asked his doctor for an honest assessment of his situation. "The doctor said, and I quote, 'If you continue, you will be a future hospital patient,'" he says.

Those weren't encouraging words, especially since Nacho's cholesterol had already been elevated for 8 years or more. With a wife and five children to think about, Nacho knew that he needed to get his cholesterol and his high blood pressure down. To spur himself into action as his 50th birthday approached, he decided to sign up for the California AIDS Bike Ride #7 the following summer—a 575-mile excursion from San Francisco to Los Angeles over a 7-day stretch.

Biking was an easy choice for Nacho, who at 5 feet 6 inches and over 300 pounds admits that he saw more activity in his youth. "Riding a bike creates no strain on your knees if the bicycle is properly set up," says this resident of Brentwood, California.

At first, Nacho rode only 12 miles a week, and he had to take a nap afterward. Eventually, he started taking short rides on weekdays and one or two longer rides on weekends. By June 2000, the month of the AIDS ride, he was covering 100 to 160 miles a week.

Training for the event spurred a number of other healthy changes as well. Nacho began drinking lots of water and juices and eating a grapefruit a day. He also gave up all fried foods.

In addition to losing 35 pounds during his training time, Nacho lowered his total cholesterol to 210 by the day of the ride. He's maintained that level to the present. "My goal is to remain consistent," he says. "I go up and down, though. It's a cross I bear every day."

But it's a cross Nacho *can* bear, thanks to how much better he feels and to the support he's received from his family, even though his training kept them apart. "They saw my energy level go up and knew it was the right thing for me to do," he says.

All of which suggests that his doctor's prognosis needs an update. Maybe something along the lines of "If he continues, he'll be a future racing champion."

WINNING ACTION

Prepare for a competition. You want to hold your own when you enter the public spotlight. If you know you're going to be squaring off against dozens, or even hundreds, of well-prepared athletes, you'll find the strength and deter-

*mination you need to get ready for the big day. You might
not bring home any medals, but your doctor and your
family will know you're a winner.*

++

NEWS FLASH: THEY'RE A STEP
AHEAD ON EXERCISE

Every morning, Mary Miner rolls out of bed at 5:15 and
switches on the news. Catching up on current events is one
way Mary likes to start her day. Walking is another. That's
why she hops on the treadmill to get her first glimpse of the
day's top stories.

Mary and her husband, Richard, bought their treadmill in
1996, while he was recuperating from a heart attack. "We
went through so much," says Mary, a 61-year-old admissions
assistant for a retirement facility in Elizabethtown, Pennsylvania. "We didn't want it to happen again."

Coincidentally, Mary had an elevated total cholesterol of
about 235, just like her husband. So she knew that whatever
lifestyle changes he made would do her heart good, too. By
walking every day and cutting her fat intake, she managed to
lower her cholesterol slightly. But it wouldn't budge below
the 200 mark.

Then in 1998, Mary learned that one of her arteries had become blocked. "Richard and I had been eating well and exercising regularly even before his heart attack," Mary says.
"Neither of us could imagine why this happened."

After undergoing coronary bypass surgery, Mary began
taking Lipitor to lower her cholesterol. (Her husband happened to be on the same medication.) She also enrolled in a
cardiac rehabilitation program for several weeks, in which
she brushed up on her nutrition information and participated in supervised exercise sessions. Her total cholesterol

plummeted to between 130 and 140, similar to her husband's.

To stay within that healthy range, the Miners pay close attention to what they're eating. They used to dine out almost every week; now they limit themselves to twice a month. At the supermarket, they buy veggie burgers instead of ground beef. And they've given up Mary's homemade, fat-filled gravies for nonfat mixes. "Most of the foods in our house are low-fat or fat-free," Mary says.

The Miners are equally meticulous about exercising regularly. After Richard's heart attack, they agreed to make time to walk every day. Since Richard had retired from his job as a pipefitter, he decided that he would walk a 2-mile loop, stopping at the local post office to pick up their mail. Mary, on the other hand, had to plan her workouts around her work schedule. That's why she resolved to get up a half-hour earlier and walk during the morning news. "I cover about a mile and a half in 25 minutes," she says.

On Saturdays, Mary gives the treadmill a rest, joining her husband on his jaunt to the post office and home again. They try to complete the 2-mile trek in 34 minutes. "By ourselves or together, we walk at least 5 days out of 7," Mary says. "We've been doing it since 1996, and we have no plans to change our routine."

WINNING ACTION

Find opportunities to walk in your daily schedule. Walking is an ideal activity for strengthening the heart muscle and lowering cholesterol. And it's easy to incorporate into even the most hectic of daily routines. You can follow Mary's lead and "multitask" by walking on the treadmill while keeping abreast of the day's news. Or you can give your walks purpose, as Richard did, by selecting a specific destination, such as the post office, pharmacy, or bank. By finding ways to add steps to your daily routine, you'll never miss a chance to keep fit.

++

SHE DITCHED THE CAR AND WALKED EVERYWHERE

In the fall of 2000, Joan Krohn's husband drove her from their home in Las Vegas, New Mexico, to the University of Illinois at Urbana-Champaign, where she had accepted a teaching assignment. Then he headed for home in the car—just as they had planned. Without transportation, Joan was forced to walk 2 to 6 miles a day—enough to shave those last stubborn points from her cholesterol.

For Joan, who's now 60, walking was an easy way to get some exercise in addition to the dance classes she took three times a week. During the fall, she rode her bike. When the winter snow hit, she switched to walking. Her office was 1 mile from her home in one direction, the grocery store a mile in another direction, and the off-campus library a mile in yet another direction. "Nothing was just outside my door," she says. "It was a real hike to get to these places."

Joan had always had good cholesterol, but around age 53, she entered menopause. She also developed hypothyroidism, which can cause cholesterol to rise. At its peak, her cholesterol reached 259, despite the fact that she was a walker and bicyclist. What's more, she followed a fairly healthy diet, with three to four servings of fruits and vegetables daily, as well as soy milk and other soy products.

Her doctor recommended taking hormone replacement therapy as a strategy to prevent osteoporosis and heart-related problems, including high cholesterol, but Joan decided to try changing her diet and getting more exercise first.

She ate even more fruits and vegetables, gave up meat in favor of fish, and left out the yolk when using eggs.

But it was an increase in walking that proved to be her most potent cholesterol remedy. In 1998, Joan spent 2½ months in Poland, researching her genealogy and living without a car. Before she left the United States, her cholesterol was at 240. Upon her return, it had dipped to 199, the lowest it's been since menopause. The next 2 years, it crept back up and hovered around 230, until she went to Urbana and gave up her car. Again, her cholesterol fell, this time to 208. "It came to me that what I was doing was being carfree," she says.

In New Mexico, Joan has had to readjust to a community with fewer sidewalks and buses, but she has adapted her exercise program. Instead of walking, she rides her bike to many destinations. And she maintains her lower cholesterol in the process.

WINNING ACTION

Get rid of your car. Or at least imagine that you don't own a car and try doing everything you can on foot, whether it's walking to the grocery store, the post office, or a friend's house. Being without a car will help you sneak in the extra exercise that just might be your key to lowering your cholesterol. It's sure to result in lost pounds, and losing weight is one of the best ways to get your cholesterol reading under control.

++

A TRIPLE BYPASS SCARED HIM INTO SHAPE

William Pensyl coached high school basketball and baseball for 40 years. Despite his enthusiasm for sports, he didn't care much for exercise. "I never enjoyed running or activities like that," confesses the 63-year-old retired teacher from Bangor, Pennsylvania.

That was before 1997, when William had to undergo a triple bypass. At the time, his cholesterol hovered around 300. Even before he left the hospital, he had made up his mind to revamp his lifestyle—and that included establishing a regular fitness program. "I was scared enough that I decided I would just do it," he recalls.

During his recovery, William participated in a hospital-sponsored rehabilitation program and read up on hospital-recommended diet and exercise plans. He literally took their advice to heart. "The day I got home, I started walking," he says. Having learned that the most beneficial fitness routine combines aerobic activity with strength training, he also decided to lift weights. He even created a schedule for himself: On Mondays, Wednesdays, and Fridays, he'd use the weight room at the high school where he had taught, and on Tuesdays, Thursdays, and Saturdays, he'd take walks. On Sundays, he'd let his body rest.

To gauge his speed while walking, William measured distances with his car odometer. "I counted my mileage by trees, figuring out which ones were $\frac{1}{10}$ of a mile apart," he says. Over the years, he has calculated countless different routes. By constantly working to go farther in less time, he is able to maintain a challenging workout. These days, he walks $4\frac{1}{2}$ miles 3 days a week—often mixing in a little jogging to pick up the pace. Even bad weather doesn't slow him down: He just drives to the high school and hops on the treadmill.

On days when he strength trains, William usually spends about 45 minutes on the various machines. "I don't lift really heavy weights, but I try to do a lot of repetitions," he says.

Right from the start, this schedule worked for William. "Alternating between walking and strength training keeps me from feeling bored," he explains. And that helps him stick with his workouts, which he's done since 1998. "I think you get to the point where if you don't exercise, you feel guilty," he says.

William has been equally committed to improving his diet. Meat, potatoes, and gravy—his former favorites—are reserved for special occasions. Now he's most likely to dine on chicken and fish. Potato chips and ice cream have vanished from his diet.

While William has been taking Lipitor—80 milligrams a day—he credits his newfound enthusiasm for exercise and eating well with improving his overall cholesterol profile. As of June 1999, his total cholesterol had dropped to 204. By January 2001, it was down to 181, with an LDL of 98, an HDL of 50, and triglycerides of 138.

By themselves, these much-improved numbers would be enough to persuade William to stick to his fitness routine. But he admits he has another reason for wanting to work out regularly: It takes him back to the school where he spent so many years teaching and coaching. "I go there every day, even if I'm just visiting," he says. "Sometimes my wife drops me off, and I walk the 4 miles home. Either way, I get in my exercise."

WINNING ACTION

For the best fitness program, mix walking and weights. From a motivational standpoint, alternating between aerobic activity and strength training can keep you from getting bored with your fitness routine. That's reason enough to try it. But switching off also ensures a well-rounded workout. While aerobic exercise gets your heart pumping and your lungs working—both essential to cardiovascular health—strength training builds muscle, which is especially important if you want to slim down and lower your cholesterol.

SHE TOOK A DIP—AND HER CHOLESTEROL SOON FOLLOWED

When Nancy A. Heeman, of Valley Stream, New York, became her mother's caregiver in 1993, she didn't expect to be nursing her husband, too. "A year later, he passed away, and I was caring for my mom on my own," she says. "I figured I'd better be in good shape."

A physical indicated that Nancy was healthy overall, while her total cholesterol level stood at 270. Her doctor told her she had to bring it down. Nancy was already walking twice a week, but she stepped it up to 1½ to 2 miles daily. "When I go out now, I have a couple of friends with me, and it becomes a nice social event," she says.

For those days when the Long Island weather doesn't cooperate, Nancy turns to her treadmill to get in her mileage.

Although the walking is enjoyable, Nancy gets a much bigger kick out of swimming. "In the summer, I swim every day at a town pool that I enjoy," she says. "I started going just out of pleasure because the water looked so inviting." When the town pool closed in September, she took to swimming for 45 minutes a couple of times a week at the high school where she works as a secretary.

Nancy has altered her diet as well, limiting herself to a teaspoon of butter per week and one or two egg whites. "In the beginning, you think this isn't quite as good, but after a while, you don't notice it," she says. "You get used to it, like going from regular bread to light bread or from regular milk to 1%."

By supplementing the swimming, walking, and diet with 10 milligrams of Lipitor daily—at her doctor's insistence—Nancy has managed to keep her total cholesterol level between 180 and 200, with an HDL level around 70. "I feel more vigorous and relatively healthy despite my age," says the 66-year-old.

She plans to retire within the next couple of years, so she's already scouting for a new swimming hole. There's a year-round pool complex not too far from her Long Island home, but that's not her only option. "I have two sons who live on the west coast of Florida," she says. "I just got back from visiting them. It's pretty darn nice to go down there in February and bask in 80-degree weather."

WINNING ACTION

Take a dip in the pool. Like walking and jogging, swimming is a full-body exercise and keeps your pulse rate elevated. But unlike those other activities, swimming is easy on the joints, which means that anyone can participate, no matter what your age or weight. Not everyone has access to the ocean, but sports clubs, YMCAs, and municipal pools offer numerous other possibilities for year-round water workouts. You might even find swimming programs at your local high school.

++

SHE SPUN THE CHOLESTEROL RIGHT OUT OF HER

In 1999, Lois Hazel got bad news from her cardiologist: Her total cholesterol reading was 232, and her triglycerides were more than 200.

Lois, 55, already had "a ghastly family history of heart disease," and she'd had high blood pressure for years. In August 1997, for example, she had a severe blood pressure spike that landed her in the emergency room. "From that time forward, I've been very conscientious about diet, exercise, and stress reduction to alleviate my hypertension," says Lois, who lives in Kintnersville, Pennsylvania.

But with high cholesterol added to the mix, she knew she

needed to do more, particularly in terms of exercise. "I'd been doing some mild aerobic activity, but not much," she says.

Lois started lifting weights and doing yoga for stress reduction, but what might have had the biggest impact was the twice-a-week Spinning class she began in late 1999. "I don't think I've ever done anything so taxing before," she says. "It's an hour long and a really tough class."

She says that Spinning was a natural for her. "I'm not very coordinated, so I don't do structured aerobics classes well," she explains. "But with the bike, I climb on and pedal to my limit. I know that I have had a wonderful workout."

What's more, on the stress test that Lois took recently, her recovery time was much faster than the year before. "I feel that the Spinning helped my endurance and recovery," she says. "My cardiologist was really pleased with the result."

In terms of her diet, Lois was already eating very little red meat and lots of fruits and vegetables, but she still found other improvements she could make. "I boosted my fiber intake, eating lots of beans, carrots, raw sunflower seeds, and bran cereal," she says. She also began drinking ginger tea at night.

By April 2001, Lois's numbers were looking a lot healthier. Her total cholesterol level had decreased to 148, with an LDL of 93 and an HDL of 35. Her triglycerides had plummeted to 102. "My family's cardiac history puts me at risk," she says. "Getting my cholesterol under control gives me one less thing to worry about."

WINNING ACTION

Sign up for a Spinning class. If you don't have the coordination or desire to bounce and step your way to aerobic success, sign up for a Spinning class at your gym, the Y, or other health club in your area. Spinning just might give you the aerobic burst you need to get your heart racing as

*well as boost your endurance, so you can last longer when
you are weight lifting, swimming, or participating in your
other favorite fitness endeavors. Since Spinning may be
more demanding than other forms of aerobic exercise,
though, consider consulting your doctor before signing up
for a class, especially if you have heart disease or several
cardiac risk factors.*

++

SHE TURNED WALKING THE DOG
INTO REAL EXERCISE

Taking the dog for a walk used to mean a quick trek around
the block for Janet Seitz. But these days, Janet and her husband, Brian, take their dog for a 3-mile jaunt around the
neighborhood and squeeze some exercise into their busy life.

Janet, a 33-year-old Portland, Oregon, resident, comes
from a family with a history of high cholesterol. "I grew up
eating low-fat, and I maintained it," she says. "I ate an apple
every day."

In her youth, exercise came naturally to her. She played
tennis from the time she was 7 and continued even through
college. But when she started her career as a retail executive,
she no longer had the time to exercise. "I do own a stationary
bike, a really nice one, but it is currently holding up boxes in
our storage unit," Janet says.

Not coincidentally, her cholesterol levels began to deterio-
rate, too. By age 29, her total cholesterol shot up to an all-
time high of 262. Family history was repeating itself, despite
Janet's healthy diet, which includes plenty of fresh fruits and
vegetables.

With a little help from Lipitor, Janet's cholesterol was
down to 189 after about a year. She quit Lipitor with plans to
get pregnant but was still concerned about her cholesterol
level.

The problem, she knew, was a lack of exercise. Working 60 hours a week and every other weekend made time a real limitation.

"One night, my husband and I decided that we—meaning the two of us and our dog—would do something as a family, and we figured that walking was the best for all of us," Janet says. "All three of us are overweight. Besides, walking gives my husband and me at least 30 minutes of quality time together to just talk. Now, we take the dog for a long walk every other day. We go about 3 miles, and we usually wind up picking up our dog before the end."

In April 2000, 6 months after she stopped taking Lipitor and a month after they started walking, Janet's cholesterol leveled out at 199. These days, the family walks every other day, rain or shine, in warm or cold. They head out after dinner and before the start of prime-time TV. They walk at least half an hour but usually go for an hour. "The fact that I can do this is a big deal," Janet says. And it's an even bigger deal now that the Seitzes are eagerly awaiting the birth of their first child.

WINNING ACTION

Take the dog for a walk. Walking Bowser is a built-in requirement for all dog owners. So why not use the chore to your own advantage? Tack some time on to the walk, add some distance, and get a proper workout. Take along your spouse or a good friend, and you'll enjoy some quality time with a companion, too. Don't have a dog of your own? Volunteer to walk a neighbor's dog, or become a volunteer dog walker for an animal shelter.

++

SHE WORKS OUT MORNING
AND NIGHT

Pat Monaghan has taken cholesterol-lowering drugs for more than a decade. And while they helped lower her numbers, she didn't achieve true success until she redoubled her exercise effort.

Back in February 1988, when Pat had her cholesterol checked at a supermarket health fair, she got a shocking result: a total cholesterol level of 320. She went on a low-fat diet at her doctor's recommendation, but when that didn't produce results, the doctor put her on Mevacor.

After 18 months on the drug, Pat developed liver problems, so her doctor switched her to a powder that's mixed with water and drunk daily. "It was terrible," says 73-year-old Pat, who lives in Philadelphia. "I could barely handle it."

But handle it she did, for 2 years. Then Zocor went on the market, and her doctor switched her to that. The new medication brought her total cholesterol level down to 220 by June 2000. At that point, Pat, who is 5 feet 2, suddenly found a bigger issue facing her: her weight of 177 pounds.

"That was an epiphany for me," says Pat. "I knew I had to do something about it." Little did she know that her weight-reduction steps would prove just as effective at lowering her cholesterol.

First on Pat's agenda was giving up all sweets. Next, she added another exercise session to her day. Now, in addition to a 2-mile walk each morning, she goes for a 20-minute walk after dinner every night ("just enough to get the metabolism moving," she says).

The absence of sweets and the extra exercise packed a solid one-two punch. By September 2000, Pat had lost 40 pounds and 60 points from her total cholesterol, bringing her to a much healthier reading of 160.

"I don't want to be fat again, and that's what motivates me now," says Pat, who also spends time caring for her 93-year-old mother—an age Pat looks forward to now that she's taking better care of herself. "I enjoy walking very much because it gives me energy for the day. I could never conceive of not walking."

‑ WINNING ACTION

Add another exercise session. Walking once a day does great things for your body, but those benefits can be undermined if you lie on the sofa the rest of the day. By adding a second exercise session—whether aerobics or biking, weight lifting or walking—you'll keep your body's metabolism revving and help drive the cholesterol from your system.

+++

GYM TIME IS TRIMMING HIS CHOLESTEROL LEVEL

George Azzopardi toted his duffel bag in and out of six gyms before he found one that suited him. "Choosing the right facility is important," explains the 50-year-old timeshare client liaison from Essex, England. "If you don't enjoy going, you give up on exercise."

Working out regularly has helped George whittle points from his total cholesterol, which in 1996 was a dangerously high 7.8 mmol/L (a British measure roughly equivalent to 300 mg/dL). "That was my wake-up call," he says. "I knew I had to do something."

Divorced and living alone, George had developed a penchant for ethnic takeout. Swearing off fast food was his first step toward lowering his cholesterol and improving his health. "I learned to cook, and my meals consisted mostly of fresh vegetables, poultry, and fish," he says. "I gave up red meats and all dairy products except skim milk." Within 6 months, his cholesterol had dropped to the mid-200s.

Encouraged, George continued with his healthy eating habits. By 1998, he had lost nearly 50 pounds, dropping his weight to its present 137. But his cholesterol seemed stuck at the same number. Determined to improve his reading, George kicked a 20-year smoking habit, an act he credits to sheer willpower. By comparison, establishing a fitness routine should have been easy. But it wasn't.

At first, George bought himself some strength-training equipment. But neither he nor the equipment got much of a workout. "I never found time to use it," he confesses. "I decided that going to a gym would be more enjoyable."

But George didn't just sign up at the nearest or most convenient facility. Instead, he checked out six different places, testing the equipment and scrutinizing the atmosphere. He realized rather quickly that none of them would cut it. "Some were too crowded. Others had old machines that didn't work well. And some didn't offer much support to their members," he explains.

Finally, in June 2000, George found the fitness center he attends today. It's a bit out of the way, and it's slightly more costly than other facilities. So what's the attraction? "This place has personal instructors who work one-on-one with clients," he says. "They help us develop and maintain our exercise schedules."

An instructor set George up with a full-body workout and tutored him on proper technique for using strength-training machines, stationary cycles, and treadmills. From the beginning, the instructor has monitored George's progress, checking his weight and modifying the workout every 4 to 6 weeks. "I like knowing that someone else is keeping an eye on what I'm doing," George says.

That extra encouragement keeps George going back to the gym on a regular basis. These days, he's working out for 2 hours, four times a week. His commitment to fitness has had a positive effect on his total cholesterol: According to his last test, it's down to 226—still higher than it should be, but oh-so-close to a healthy range.

WINNING ACTION

Choose a gym that you're comfortable with. Investing in a gym membership may provide extra incentive to start and stick with an exercise program. Just make sure the facility can accommodate your interests and lifestyle. You may prefer a place close to home, or with flexible hours, or with a wide variety of classes and equipment. Decide which factors are most important to you, then shop around. Once you find the right place and establish a fitness routine, you'll see a positive change in your cholesterol profile (not to mention your weight!).

++

AT THE GYM, SHE COUNTS ON THE BUDDY SYSTEM

Every morning, Barbara Barber looks forward to a chat with a friend. But she never picks up the phone. Instead, she laces her sneakers and heads for the gym. She spends an hour and a half working out and conversing with the other women there.

"When I'm on the treadmill and I'm talking with the person next to me, time just flies by," says Barbara, a 49-year-old Rome, New York, resident who works with the mentally challenged. The conversation and camaraderie keep her going back to the gym on a daily basis—and helped her lower her cholesterol by more than 130 points.

It took a serious health crisis to convince her to start exercising in the first place. One evening in 1994, Barbara, then a full-time mother of three, fell ill with severe back pain and nausea. She went to her doctor 2 days later, hoping to find out what was wrong. She thought she had a bad case of the flu. The diagnosis stunned her: She had had a severe heart attack.

"I felt completely devastated," Barbara recalls. "I became convinced that my life was over, and that I'd never be the same again."

As she would learn later, an inherited tendency toward high cholesterol, coupled with an unhealthy lifestyle, had put her at grave risk. "Back then, I was overweight, smoking a pack and a half a day, and not eating properly," she says. "I wasn't thinking about my health. Being a mother, I was too busy taking care of everyone else."

And it showed: Her total cholesterol had reached a sky-high 280, and her triglycerides hovered between 500 and 600. She also learned that she had developed type 2 (non-insulin-dependent) diabetes.

But the heart attack was the real wake-up call. It left Barbara without the function of two-thirds of her heart muscle.

Immediately, Barbara quit smoking, gave up sweets and red meat, and switched to fruits, vegetables, whole grains, and low-fat dairy products. She also launched a fitness routine, starting with daily ½-mile walks to facilitate her recovery. "The heart attack did a lot of damage, so I had to go really slow," she says. "Most days I split my workout in half, so I could rest in between."

Within 7 months, Barbara was walking 2 to 3 miles a day. All the while, her total cholesterol was sliding downward.

Despite her transformed lifestyle, Barbara developed another blockage in her arteries. In 1999, she underwent a triple coronary bypass. Even after the surgery, her total cholesterol and triglycerides were 210 and 395, respectively. "My doctors gave me a prescription for Lipitor to help modify my hereditary tendency toward high cholesterol," she explains.

That's when her son, Josh, intervened. "With winter approaching, he suggested that we join a gym," Barbara says. "That way, I could work out every day, even in cold or rainy weather. He showed me some strength-training exercises and explained all the machines. Once I got started, it was easy and enjoyable."

Barbara soon realized that the gym offered more than protection from the elements. "I got to know a number of women there, and we'd talk while we worked out," she says. "That made me look forward to my exercise sessions."

Those workouts helped Barbara's heart health tremendously. Within several months, her total cholesterol dropped to 145, and her triglycerides to 125. Both measures have stayed solidly within a healthy range ever since.

Even though her cholesterol profile has improved dramatically, Barbara hasn't given up her gym routine. These days, her workouts consist of a 3-mile walk on the treadmill, a 5-mile spin on the stationary cycle, and upper- and lower-body strength training on the weight machines on alternating days. It's physically challenging, but Barbara enjoys every minute of it. "Exercising with others seems to make my routine much more pleasant and easier," she says. "Still, I never forget that the changes I have made in my lifestyle are for *me*. They are for life."

WINNING ACTION

Find a fitness partner at the local gym. Having someone to work out with can make a big difference in the long-term success of your exercise program. But what if your spouse doesn't enjoy the same activity as you do, or your neighbor isn't free to go walking when you are? Then you have all the more reason to join a gym. No matter when *you're there, you'll meet people who can keep you company and help the time fly. Pretty soon, your workouts will seem less like work and more like a chance to socialize. That can be good for your heart, too!*

++

HE STARTED RUNNING AND NEVER LOOKED BACK

In 1993, Michael Griffin was a textbook case of heart disease risks: 65 pounds overweight and a 3-decade smoker, with a father who had died of a heart attack at age 49 and two uncles who had died similarly before age 60.

The final red flag was a total cholesterol reading of 315, but he didn't recognize it—until his heart attack in February of that year. Then, Michael says, "I worked to undergo a complete lifestyle change."

Michael, a 52-year-old high school sociology teacher from Janesville, Wisconsin, began walking, then jogging, then running. "I quickly became addicted to the positive motivation, fellowship, and physical and emotional high I received from being around other runners—the most positive group of people I have ever met," he says.

But running gave him more than just positive feelings. "As my endurance increased and my pace quickened, I began to increase my mileage to 2 to 3 miles per day," says Michael. "When I increased my mileage to 5 to 6 miles each morning before school, I decided to enter a number of noncompetitive fun runs in the area."

While competing in the fun runs, Michael realized he was in much better shape than he'd thought. "I decided to enter a 5-K race and then a number of 10-Ks," he says. "In short order, I ran a 10-miler and then graduated to my first half-marathon. In May of 1994, I entered the Madison Marathon. Finishing in less than 4 hours, I was addicted." Since then, he's completed eight more marathons, including ones in Chicago, Boston, and Las Vegas.

As he progressed, Michael created running-related goals—distances, times, frequency—to keep him motivated. "Another goal of mine is to someday be able to run a 10-K event or longer with my granddaughter, Alex (now 8), and my grandson, Will (now 2)," he says.

In addition to becoming a long-distance runner, Michael reduced his fat consumption to 10 percent of his total calories. "I was on the classic 'see-food' diet. Whatever I saw, I ate," he says. "My diet now consists of vegetables, fruits, grains, and a small amount of fish, chicken, or turkey."

Through diet and exercise, Michael, at 5 feet 8 inches tall, went from 225 pounds to 160, and his cholesterol figures became ideal. In May 2000, his total cholesterol level was 174, his LDL level was 100, and his ratio (a comparison of total cholesterol to HDL) was a sparkling 3.2:1. "If I can continue to put in the hard work necessary to maintain a healthy and vibrant lifestyle, the future is bright and, hopefully, long," he says. And for now, "I've kept the weight off and feel like a new human being."

WINNING ACTION

Run—and the world runs with you. There are any number of events that you can participate in if running is your chosen exercise. In fun runs, your fellow runners will spur you on to success, encouraging you to keep exercising and improving. Even if you don't win the race, you still come out on top by losing weight and maintaining the motivation to stick with a cholesterol-lowering fitness program.

++

A LITTLE MUSIC MAKES
WALKING MORE INTERESTING

When Paul Minor first started walking, he found his mind swimming with thoughts of what else he could be doing, be it something on the computer or watching TV. Then he started using a digital tape player with classical music, and his walks became more gratifying and productive.

"Music occupies my mind, and time becomes less of a factor," says Paul, a 61-year-old dentist from Forest Grove, Oregon. "It's a mental diversion."

Paul took up walking in 1999, when doctors discovered he had diabetes, and high cholesterol along with it. His cholesterol at the time was 300. Paul had been feeling tired, and his left foot hurt, symptoms of diabetes that he initially ignored, until he started urinating more frequently and feeling more thirsty. Discovering he had high cholesterol was a by-product of his diagnosis for diabetes.

As part of his initial treatment for both problems, Paul decided to follow an eating plan that advocated more proteins and fewer carbohydrates. In particular, he cut back on grain products and increased his consumption of meats, fish, dairy products (except milk and yogurt), and vegetables—especially broccoli, cauliflower, cabbage, peppers, salad greens, and onions. While a low-carbohydrate diet is not often recommended, Paul feels he couldn't have reined in his cholesterol or blood sugar without it.

To supplement his dietary changes, Paul took up walking, usually with his dog. He started by walking 30 minutes on level surfaces in his neighborhood. Over time, as his stamina grew, he started walking for longer periods and tackling more hills. "The hills get your heart pumping and your breathing going," he says. "Now I go up and down two fairly big hills, and if I feel more energetic, I might go up three or four times."

But Paul, who sings in a few choirs, wanted to do more

than walk. Friends of his listened to ballgames or motivational tapes while they exercised. Paul decided to take along tapes of classical music, recordings by his choir, and even his own solos. "You gain insight into hearing yourself sing," he says. "It gives you feedback, and it's a lot different from having a coach tell you what to do."

While Paul credits his dietary changes with making the biggest dent in his cholesterol, as well as his blood sugar, he knows that his walking program has played a role, too. Over the course of 3 months, his cholesterol fell to 271. When he gave up his four daily egg yolks, his total cholesterol dropped to 194, while his HDL level soared. Sticking with his diet-and-exercise regimen has kept his cholesterol profile in excellent shape.

These days, Paul walks two or three evenings a week for about 45 minutes each time, and on the weekends, he walks in the morning. He has lost about 15 pounds, dropping to 150 pounds on his 5-foot-10 frame. More important to Paul, he's controlling his diabetes without medication. "Managing my blood sugar keeps me motivated," he says.

WINNING ACTION

Listen to music or other kinds of tapes while you walk. Tapes provide an entertaining distraction from the mere act of walking or doing other exercises. They also help while away the time if you're prone to boredom. For safety reasons, make sure you can hear what's going on around you. That's especially important if you're walking in traffic areas.

++

GARDENING PLANTED THE SEEDS
OF GOOD HEALTH

"Some call me the farmer, and some call me the tomato man," says Edmund Reybitz. And with good reason.

Edmund, 79, puts out over 100 tomato plants every year. He stakes each one and, once they start producing, gathers their fruit every day.

"I keep my family, friends, and neighbors supplied," he says. "I take tomatoes to the nuns every week, and to our priest."

Edmund plants several varieties of tomatoes, including two types of red, a yellow, and a miniature grape. He also grows yellow string beans, peppers, yellow and green zucchini squash, and a variety of flowers—all started from seed. His garden thrives on the grounds of Kirkland Village, a senior community in Bethlehem, Pennsylvania, where Edmund and his wife, Claire, who has Alzheimer's disease, reside.

"Gardening occupies my mind," Edmund says. "It is my incentive, my motivation, to stay healthy." In fact, combined with a healthy diet and medication, gardening helps hold his cholesterol level below 150.

In 1996, Edmund had a heart attack. After that, his doctor prescribed Lescol, a cholesterol-lowering drug.

In May 2000, Edmund's total cholesterol was 180, with an HDL of 33 and an LDL of 134. But his doctor, concerned about the possibility of a second heart attack, wasn't satisfied. He changed Edmund's medicine to Lipitor. And then he asked Edmund about his diet.

"I was eating ice cream every night," Edmund says. "And cheese melts: I was making them at lunch. The doctor said, 'You're going to have to cut out that stuff.'"

And cut it out he did. "I stopped eating them that day," Edmund says. "It wasn't hard." He replaced the cheese melts with cereal and fruit; he eliminated the evening ice cream snack completely.

"He is a very determined person," says Edmund's daughter, Barbara. "He is determined to be healthy. He wants to be able to work in the garden."

At his visit to the doctor in July 2000, Edmund's total cholesterol had dropped to an amazing 112. His LDL was 62 and his HDL 41.

In addition, he had dropped 23 pounds. At 6 feet 2, he had gone from 228 to 205.

Edmund says that he is proud of his cholesterol level. He is also proud of his 150-square-foot garden. He started gardening in 1992, after bad knees put a halt to his four-times-a-week golf game. Now during gardening season, his plants keep him so busy that he often doesn't have time for his usual half-hour workout at the on-site gym.

Since he and his wife moved into Kirkland Village in 1997, Edmund has obtained permission to use part of his apartment building's basement to start seeds for his garden. Despite having undergone a knee replacement, he is planning to grow all his traditional vegetables and flowers as well as to expand into spinach.

In 2000, he grew pumpkins for the first time. On Thanksgiving, he surprised his family with a pumpkin pie he had baked. "It was really good," he says. "And I enjoyed making it. When you have a garden, there is always something new to do."

WINNING ACTION

Take up gardening. Tilling, planting, weeding, and cultivating all get your heart pumping, which helps keep it strong. Gardening by necessity is done outside and brings you closer to all forms of life, from the lowly earthworm to the neighbors dropping by for a few tomatoes. And there is little that is as life-affirming as watching a tiny brown seed sprout, grow into a vibrant plant, and produce a good-for-you harvest.

++

A LITTLE VARIETY SPICED UP
HIS WORKOUTS

Lifelong runners like Roy Bragger tend to have little patience for walking. So when a heart attack forced Roy to slow his pace, he made his walks more interesting by varying his routes.

Having been a competitive runner for most of his adult life, Roy was accustomed to an active lifestyle. That changed in 1993, when he developed liver disease and underwent a liver transplant. As a result of his illness, Roy dropped 45 pounds from his already lean 5-foot-8-inch frame in about 9 months. To get back to 150 pounds, he filled up on beef, eggs, and cheese—cholesterol-laden foods that he had always eaten with reckless abandon.

In October 1994, while trying to resume his running regimen, Roy had a massive heart attack. His cholesterol had hit an all-time high of 348. "Genetics probably played a role, as did my diet," says the 71-year-old Syracuse, New York, resident. "When I stopped running, these other risk factors caught up with me."

To get back in shape after his heart attack and subsequent quadruple bypass surgery, Roy had to take small steps—a challenge for the native Briton, who was accustomed to running. He started by walking from his home to the corner of his block and back, a distance of ¼ mile. Eventually, he could go around the entire block, a full ½ mile. "I remember feeling pretty proud when I could walk a mile and a half without sitting down," he says.

Still, walking isn't the same as running. "I didn't get the same satisfaction from walking as from running. I didn't get that 'runner's high,'" Roy says. "Walking just takes longer, too."

To make his workouts more stimulating, Roy varied his routes. One day he would walk along a country road dotted by farms. The next he'd meet up with his walking buddy, a little boy who'd keep him company for part of his route.

Sometimes he ventured into unfamiliar neighborhoods to check out the homes under construction. Other times he headed for the grocery store or a nearby lake. "By mixing up my routes, walking became more interesting," Roy says. "Going the same direction all the time can get a bit stale."

When winter arrived, Roy joined the local YMCA so he could walk indoors. He also did some strength training. To shape up his eating habits, he cut back on red meat, eggs, and dairy products. Eighteen months after having heart surgery, his cholesterol had fallen to 150.

Since then, Roy—to satisfy his competitive spirit—has taken up racewalking. In 1997, he won two medals for race-walking in New York's Empire State Senior Games. When he's not training, he works as a personal trainer for the YMCA and participates in local fund-raising walks. Not bad for a guy who thought walking wasn't his cup of tea!

WINNING ACTION

Change your workout. No matter how much you may enjoy exercising, doing the same thing day after day (after day) can become tedious. And that can quickly sap your motivation. Look for ways to add some variety to your workouts. If you're walking, for example, change your routes. If you're strength training, try adding intervals of aerobic activity to your routine. Even minor changes like these can help keep your fitness regimen on track.

++

A DAILY DOSE OF EXERCISE KEEPS HER BODY RUNNING

Ellen Mazo, 53, of Emmaus, Pennsylvania, has been a runner for half her life—but running by itself doesn't guarantee perfect health. In 1992, for example, her total cholesterol level was 205, despite a 15-year running habit that included a half-dozen marathons.

What's more, Ellen knew that women going through menopause typically see their cholesterol numbers go up. That was something she couldn't accept, so she decided to participate in a randomized clinical trial at the University of Pittsburgh Graduate School of Public Health. Researchers there were trying to show that healthy women going through menopause could keep their LDL cholesterol and weight down.

"They worked with me to change my whole pattern of eating, so I'd limit my cholesterol intake to 100 milligrams a day, my calories to around 1,500 a day, my total fat intake to 25 percent of calories, and my saturated fat intake to 7 percent of calories," says Ellen. "I even increased my exercise level. And it worked. I've been following the same program since 1992, and I'm very happy with it."

In terms of her diet, Ellen says that she's much more aware of food labels, fat content, portion size, and her total intake. "I cut out desserts like cookies, cakes, and pies completely, even if someone makes a homemade pie," she says. "If I crave sweets, I'll eat something nonfat like jelly beans."

As for the exercise, Ellen decided to copy the success she'd had with running and added walking to her schedule. "When I started in 1977, I ran a mile a day, 6 days a week," she says. "I lifted weights and did other exercise but not consistently like the running. The running took only 10 minutes a day, so I knew I could do that."

Ellen ran a mile a day for 2 years, then found a 3-mile track and started on that. "That was a half-hour each day, and I knew I could do it," she says. After a few more years, she ran her first 10-K race and then a marathon. "But no matter what, in all those years, I'd do at least a mile a day," she says.

In 1992, as part of the study, she began walking 2 miles a day on top of the running, and she noticed immediate changes. "My weight stabilizes when I include walking," says Ellen. "When you train for marathons, you get really hungry and eat more; the walking helps use up those calories without tiring you out."

Now, long after the study's end, Ellen maintains her cholesterol-lowering ways and has kept her total cholesterol level between 160 and 170 consistently. "As dedicated as I am to running, I'm convinced that a regular regimen of walking at least 2 miles a day is key," says Ellen. "If you can't run, at least walk. You have to find something you can fit in, even if you feel you have no time at all."

WINNING ACTION

Create an exercise routine you can do consistently. The most important part of exercise isn't the number of pounds you lift, the lengths you swim, or the miles you run, but the fact that you do it on a regular basis. Regular bouts of exercise keep your body running on an even keel and give you confidence to keep improving because you know that you're always making progress.

++

THE GOAL OF GOOD HEALTH KEEPS HIM GOING

John Lynch isn't a big fan of exercise. "I'd rather do just about anything else," he confesses. "Motivation doesn't come easily to me."

Still, John knows that staying fit and eating well are vital to his long-term heart health. So he sticks with them. And if his desire starts to flag, he remembers the words of one particular cardiac rehabilitation nurse. "I was complaining about having to exercise," he recalls. "She said to me, 'John, you don't have to *like* it. Just *do* it!' "

As you might imagine, John—a 71-year-old retired airline pilot from Laguna Hills, California—didn't always take good care of himself. He might not have changed his unhealthy ways were it not for a stress test in 1987. He remembers it well. "I had been on the treadmill for about 30 seconds when the doctor stopped me and handed me a nitroglycerin tablet to put under my tongue," he says. "He was actually shaking, although I didn't notice anything unusual."

In fact, John had two blocked coronary arteries that required angioplasty. Before that, a blood test had showed his total cholesterol to be around 285, increasing his risk of a heart attack. Six months after the stress test, John underwent another angioplasty after his doctor determined that the first one didn't take.

Postsurgery, John enrolled in a 3-month cardiac rehabilitation program. He attended classes on nutrition, lifestyle, and stress management, and participated in closely monitored exercise sessions—aerobic activity and strength training—for 1 hour three times a week. Based on his own research, John also began taking niacin.

Through the 3 months of the program, John's total cholesterol dropped to an acceptable level. Then he was on his own, though he continued to have his cholesterol checked every month for about 18 months. "From those blood tests, I realized that if I neglected any one of the three components of my program—diet, exercise, or niacin—my cholesterol would climb," he says.

So John continuously prodded himself to follow all he had learned during his 3-month stint in cardiac rehabilitation (which he repeated 2 years later as a refresher). He built his meals around high-fiber, low-fat foods, starting every day with a breakfast of oat bran, fruit, and fat-free milk. He resisted the urge to indulge in doughnuts and sugary snacks. And three times a week, he rode a stationary cycle and lifted weights, either at home or at a gym.

Even old injuries to his knee and ankle didn't completely discourage John from working out, though they did slow him down. "Because of my knee, I couldn't pedal too vigorously, especially uphill," he says. "And my ankle kept me from walking for more than an hour at a time. Cycling outdoors and walking for long distances were out of the question."

That was enough to start John's cholesterol inching upward. So in 1997, his doctor took him off niacin and put him on Zocor, which he continues taking today. According to his latest test, his total cholesterol stands at a very healthy 144.

John could easily let the medication do the work and give up on his lifestyle changes. But he has no intention of doing so. "I've had to accept that I have a medical condition, and that a healthy lifestyle is a necessity for my condition," he says. "I know that my future depends on my actions now. If I take care of myself, my reward will be a longer and happier life. If I don't take care of myself, I'll die before I need to. It's that simple."

WINNING ACTION

Do what you need to. To bring your cholesterol to a healthy level, you may find yourself adopting strategies that you don't necessarily enjoy. Rather than finding reasons not to follow through on them, remind yourself why you should. Then do whatever you must to make those strategies stick. If you really dislike exercise, for example, promise yourself some postworkout pampering by soaking in a warm bath or watching your favorite TV show. That may give you a little incentive to work out. So may the long-term reward: a longer, healthier life.

++

GET THE NUMBERS YOU
WANT NATURALLY

✦ ✦ ✦

SHE HIRED PROFESSIONALS
TO HELP HER MEET HER GOALS

Rosanne Paschal, 51, had quite a shock when her doctor ran a series of tests in January 1999. This resident of Naperville, Illinois, already knew she had a problem with her cholesterol; it had been as high as 320 in the past. But she also discovered that she had high blood pressure plus high levels of lipids, uric acid, and sugar. "It scared the life out of me," she says. "I imagined myself getting diabetes."

The doctor prescribed Lipitor for her cholesterol, but Rosanne knew that she needed some serious help. Instead of taking matters into her own hands, she decided to go the professional route. The first thing she did was to visit a registered dietitian. The dietitian put her on a 1,400-calorie diet that reduced carbs, sugar, and fat. She also educated Rosanne about fats, especially trans fats. "I switched to good fats, drank fat-free instead of whole milk, and ate more fruits and vegetables," she says. "I also cut down on egg yolks. Now my absolute favorite is an egg white omelette."

Rosanne became an avid label reader and kept a food log at the recommendation of the R.D. "I don't buy anything unless I read it first," she says. And while she was refurbishing her eating habits, Rosanne's regular appointments with the dietitian provided her with inspiration and education.

At about the same time, Rosanne started working with a degreed and certified personal trainer, who guided her through 50-minute exercise sessions three days a week. Her program consisted of a cardiovascular workout on a recumbent bicycle, treadmill, and StairMaster, as well as flexibility and strength training through resistance exercises and weight lifting.

Within 6 months, thanks to the help of these health professionals, Rosanne's cholesterol level dropped to 197. By November 2000, her body mass index (which helps assess disease risk) went from over 50 to a much healthier 29, and her body fat percentage decreased from 50 percent to 28 percent. And within a year and a half, she lost an amazing 120 pounds. Says Rosanne, "I feel energized. People say I look younger. I feel happy."

WINNING ACTION

Team up with a registered dietitian and other health professionals. If fighting the cholesterol war is too overwhelming or if you don't know where to start, take your woes to a health professional. A dietitian will customize a diet for you and educate you on healthy eating. A personal trainer will create an exercise program for your individual needs. To find a dietitian in your area, visit the American Dietetic Association's Web site at www.eatright.org and enter your zip code in the box. To find a personal trainer, contact a fitness center or YMCA.

++

HE KEPT MAKING CHANGES—AND HIS NUMBERS KEPT FALLING

Wayne Morrow always imagined himself as fairly healthy. He ate lots of fruits, vegetables, and tofu. He exercised often. He never smoked. Despite his best efforts, though, his body seemed to have other ideas.

In 1994, after his total cholesterol level had reached 265, Wayne—an engineer from Boulder, Colorado—had a heart attack. He never thought it would happen to him. During his recovery, he made up his mind to find out what had gone wrong and what he needed to do differently.

First, he went through Boulder Community Hospital's 6-week cardiac rehabilitation program, which was based on Dr. Dean Ornish's Program for Reversing Heart Disease. Among other things, he realized that his old diet—the one he considered nutritious—actually contained a lot of fast-food lunches and no special limitation on fat.

One of the first changes Wayne made was to reduce his fat intake in accordance with the Ornish program. That was enough to shave 50 points from his total cholesterol, dropping it to 210 in just 4 months. Encouraged, Wayne believed he could do even better.

He started visiting his health club almost daily, taking classes in Spinning—a specialized form of stationary cycling—3 days a week. The rest of his time was split between weight lifting and yoga classes. "I probably exercise twice as much as before," he says. He also enjoyed cycling and skiing cross-country with his family.

His improved diet and increased physical activity, combined with a modest dose of Zocor, reduced his total cholesterol to 175 and his weight to 162—a loss of 20 pounds from his 5-foot-9 frame. "I got rid of all the bulges, and I've maintained my weight and my fitness level," he says.

After 5 years of a low-fat, mostly vegetarian diet, Wayne began eating more fish to increase his intake of heart-healthy omega-3 fatty acids. For the same reason, he added flaxseed oil to his diet, choosing to avoid oils high in saturated fats. "It's all part of the process of learning which foods to eat and which to avoid," he explains. With each of these changes, his cholesterol dropped a little more.

Today, at age 53, Wayne sports an enviable total cholesterol level of 170, which he achieved within 2 months of going on Zocor. But that's not what he's most proud of. He's thrilled that his recovery has sparked lifestyle changes in the people around him. "My wife and daughter went on diets similar to mine, and they got great benefits from it," Wayne says. "My daughter's lost weight and lowered her cholesterol, and my wife gained a healthier perspective about the impact of food and food preparation on our family's health."

WINNING ACTION

Don't limit yourself to only one solution. Dropping beef from your diet will lower your fat intake, and adding an extra exercise session will help keep you fit. But you can always do more to lower your cholesterol. Even minor lifestyle changes can add up to major improvements in your numbers. Switch from white bread to whole grain. Use flaxseed oil instead of hydrogenated ones. While watching TV, do stretches rather than lying on the sofa. When you integrate multiple cholesterol-fighting strategies into your life, you'll have an even better chance of keeping your heart strong!

HE DROPPED THE CIGARETTES, AND HIS CHOLESTEROL

Bruce Krafft knew he was at risk for heart disease, but he never got beyond the "intention" stage of doing something about it. This 39-year-old resident of Maplewood, Minnesota, had been smoking for 15 years and was 50 to 100 pounds overweight for at least that long. As of June 1999, his total cholesterol level was 280, his HDL level 23, and his triglyceride reading over 600.

Everything changed at 3:30 A.M. on April 16, 2000. How does Bruce remember that date so clearly? "I was driving home from an after-dancing supper when the back pain that had started at the restaurant ran around to my chest and began shooting down my left arm and up into my jaw," he says.

By chance, he was passing a hospital, so he pulled into the emergency room. "By the time I got to the ER desk, the pain was so bad I could hardly see," says Bruce. "After they took an EKG, they were literally passing it around the ER saying, 'See? This is what a heart attack looks like in the first 30 minutes.' "

The cigarette Bruce smoked on his way to the hospital turned out to be his last. Suddenly, kicking the habit seemed quite easy. "I had no problem quitting smoking as I was lying in the cardiac intensive care unit awaiting quadruple bypass surgery," he says. "But I would have been much better off doing it so much earlier."

In addition to dropping the butts, Bruce eliminated butter from his diet. "I have jam on my toast and bagels and use canola oil or olive oil with a bit of salt in recipes that call for butter," he says. "I don't even use margarine or any other butter substitutes."

That's quite a change from his old eating habits. "I used to go through more than a pound of butter a week," says Bruce, mentioning that he would eat "a bagel with half a stick of butter on it as a snack." He also cut out eggs and almost all red meat, eating fish, chicken, or vegetarian dishes instead.

Along with making changes in his diet, Bruce launched a walking program. At first, he did 10-minute workouts a few times a day. Eventually, he was able to walk for an hour straight.

By June 2000, Bruce's cholesterol numbers were shining: total 142, LDL 74, HDL 45, and triglycerides 113. His weight also improved, going from 320 to 270 on his 6-foot-5 frame.

After experiencing Bruce's heart attack and seeing the great progress that he's made, his father and four older siblings started eating better and exercising. "As my sister pointed out, 'Because of you, we now have a family history of heart disease,'" he says.

And with the positive changes to his own life, Bruce is determined to make his bypass last for 20 years.

WINNING ACTION

Stop smoking. A smoker is more than twice as likely as a nonsmoker to have a heart attack, and the risk of sudden cardiac death is up to four times as high. No one ever says it's easy to quit smoking, but it makes a lot more sense to quit now than to hope that you still have a chance to quit once you're lying in the hospital bed. Talk to your doctor about ways to kick the habit.

++

A B VITAMIN IS HIS CHOLESTEROL BUSTER OF CHOICE

Eighty-one-year-old Herman Arrow can walk circles around many people half his age. He's a racewalker, one of about 10 athletes competing nationally in the same age bracket.

His achievement is especially impressive considering that in 1986, Herman—a former wine industry sales manager from Greenbrae, California—was recovering from a quadruple bypass. He hadn't engaged in a formal exercise program since high school. These days, he trains for an hour 6 days a week.

Racewalking has helped Herman reduce his cholesterol to a safe level. So has following a strict diet of plant foods, with an occasional serving of fish. But ask Herman how his heart-healthy lifestyle got its start, and he might mention a certain supplement: niacin, one of the B vitamins.

Soon after he had his surgery, Herman was given a prescription for medication to help lower his total cholesterol from an unhealthful 250. But he really didn't like the idea of taking drugs, possibly for life.

A few months later, Herman came across an article about niacin in a health journal. "I showed the article to my doctor, and he said, 'Try it and see if it works,' " Herman recalls. So he did, replacing his medication with 500 milligrams of niacin a day. "It definitely made a difference," he says.

After another few months, encouraged by the results, Herman increased his dosage by 500 milligrams. That dropped his total cholesterol even farther, to between 150 and 175.

Herman admits that niacin had its drawbacks. At first, he was bothered by the supplement's well-known flushing effect, brought on by the dilation of blood vessels in the skin. "You kind of burn up for 15 minutes, then cool down," he says. "A lot of people don't like it." He put up with it for a year before switching to timed-release niacin. That put an end to the unpleasant reaction.

Soon after, a blood test showed an increase in Herman's liver enzymes, another of niacin's common side effects. "My doctor wanted me to stop taking niacin altogether," Herman says. "Instead, I went to a holistic nutritionist, who suggested that I try a B-vitamin complex, often referred to as super-B complex." He took the nutritionist's advice, and within several months, his liver enzymes had returned to normal.

Herman still takes his super-B complex, along with a new flush-free form of niacin that doesn't affect his liver. According to his most recent screening, his total cholesterol is holding steady at 165 to 175. His overall cholesterol profile is looking good, too: HDL, 55; LDL, 95; and triglycerides, 135.

"In itself, niacin isn't a panacea," stresses Herman, who has served as president of his local Mended Hearts chapter (affiliated with the American Heart Association) since 1988. "If you don't make other changes, like eating better and exercising more, it won't work as well." He believes that niacin, as part of an overall healthy lifestyle, can be effective.

WINNING ACTION

Ask your doctor about niacin supplements. Studies have shown that niacin can effectively lower total cholesterol and triglycerides. But because it must be taken in very large doses, it must be done under medical supervision. If one form of niacin raises liver enzymes, your doctor can help you find another that works better for you.

++

SO FAR, SOY'S GOOD

When Dorothy DeLabar's cholesterol plummeted from 290 to 165 in just 6 weeks, perhaps no one was as thrilled as she was. But her excitement was tempered by concern that she might need to give up her treatment of choice: soy protein.

Dorothy learned that she had cholesterol trouble in September 1999. Besides a high total reading, she had very high LDL (199) and high triglycerides (289). She decided to try a soy protein supplement powder after reading that it had shown benefit as a cholesterol treatment. Now Dorothy was reading controversial reports that women who've had breast cancer shouldn't use soy protein. It contains plant estrogens, or phytoestrogens, which a few experts believe could increase the risk of recurrence. A dozen years earlier, in 1987, Dorothy had been diagnosed with breast cancer and had undergone a mastectomy.

Dorothy—a nurse herself—asked a nurse in her gynecologist's office whether she could continue using soy protein. The nurse assured her that the supplement was safe, but her gynecologist wasn't so sure. "She told me that some say it's safe, while others say it isn't," recalls Dorothy, a 65-year-old Easton, Pennsylvania, resident. "So in early 2000, I stopped taking it. I switched to soy milk and tofu because I'd heard that their plant estrogens aren't as concentrated."

She made other changes in her diet as well, giving up beef and ice cream—both high in fat—and cutting back on chicken and fish to three or four servings a week. At the same time, she increased her consumption of fresh fruit and vegetables—her favorites are cantaloupes, grapes, tomatoes, and sweet potatoes—and whole grains. She also started walking 3 miles a day.

Despite these efforts, her total cholesterol rose from 165 to 215 within 6 weeks after she stopped using soy protein. By October 2000, it was up to 226. That convinced her to go back to her supplement powder.

"I did more reading, and I talked twice with the surgeon who does my mastectomy checkups. I felt completely comfortable with my decision to resume using soy protein," she says. "After all, some doctors think you shouldn't take vitamins, but others think you should take megadoses. You need to make the best decision for yourself."

Dorothy takes two 11-gram scoops of soy protein a day. In the morning, she whips a vanilla-flavored powder into 10 ounces of orange juice. "It's a little thick, but I've gotten used to it," she says.

On cool nights, before going to bed, Dorothy warms up a cup of fat-free milk, then stirs in a scoop of chocolate-flavored soy protein powder. "I like to think of it as hot chocolate," she says. In warmer weather, she uses cold milk to make her version of chocolate milk. Both beverages taste like the real thing, she says.

She spends about $9 a week on her soy protein products, but

Dorothy thinks it's money well-spent. And she has a cholesterol reading to back her up. According to her most recent test, her total cholesterol has dropped to 190, with LDL at 127. Her triglycerides, while still high at 203, have also improved. As a bonus, she has lost 15 pounds; at 5 feet 5, she's down to 150. "Because the soy protein contains 108 calories per scoop, I suspect some of my other dietary changes—like giving up ice cream—have helped compensate for it," she says.

Dorothy hopes her cholesterol will drop even lower. Right now, she's just grateful that it's under control. "My doctor said he would put me on medication if I didn't reduce my cholesterol within 3 months," she says. "I'm very sensitive to medicine; I tend to have a lot of side effects. Anything I can do to avoid drugs, I'll do. I want to live to a ripe old age and be around to enjoy my great-grandchildren."

WINNING ACTION

Try taking soy as a supplement. Haven't developed a taste for tofu or the other soy foods on the market? You can still get your soy protein in supplement form. According to the FDA, eating 25 grams (just under 1 ounce) of soy protein a day—in combination with an otherwise healthy diet—can help lower the risk of heart disease. Research has linked certain compounds in soy protein, called isoflavones, with reduced blood cholesterol. You can find soy protein products in health food stores.

SHE ADDED FAT TO HER DIET—AND LOWERED HER CHOLESTEROL

As CEO of LaCrista, a natural skin care company, Linda Collinson has spent a lot of time educating herself about natural approaches to health. She knows that eating the right kind of fat is just as important as monitoring your total fat intake.

She got a reminder of this lesson in 2000, when, around the time she turned 50, she read through the risk factors that women encounter as they get older. "I knew that I needed to keep my risks low," says Linda, who lives in Annapolis, Maryland. "The older you get, the more the risks hit home."

Linda had already lowered her cholesterol from 290 to 250 by taking medication for her hypothyroidism. But her HDL level was 40, and she knew that her heart attack risk would decrease with a higher reading. Drawing on her background in natural remedies, she added nutrients like niacin, vitamin C, vitamin E, and B-complex vitamins to her diet as well as more fiber.

"I also added more of the right types of fat to my diet: evening primrose oil and flaxseed oil, which lower triglycerides and raise HDL cholesterol," says Linda. "Since I usually work long hours and seldom cook, I bought flaxseed oil in the bottle, and I take a teaspoon of the oil daily along with five gel-caps of evening primrose oil."

By making these changes in her diet and adding weight lifting and treadmill work three times a week, Linda was able to bring her total cholesterol level down to 219 and boost her HDL level to 61. What's more, she has been able to pass on what she's learned, which means that her children probably won't wait until middle age to start watching their numbers. Says Linda, "My kids are much more aware of health and healthy living than I was at their age."

WINNING ACTION

Get the right types of fat with primrose oil and flaxseed oil. Totally eliminating fat from your diet isn't possible, or even a goal worth attempting. While foods like meat, eggs, but-

*ter, many vegetable oils, and margarine contribute to rais-
ing LDL cholesterol, other fats like primrose and flaxseed
oils contain essential fatty acids that may help increase
beneficial HDL cholesterol.*

++

HE FINDS WINE MORE THAN
A RELAXING DRINK

Stephen Adams's doctor had two pieces of advice for attacking a cholesterol level of 241: Exercise regularly and add red
wine to the daily dinner menu. Stephen was already swimming and playing basketball, so he decided to start drinking a
single 4-ounce glass of red wine with his evening meal. Sure
enough, the next time he had his cholesterol checked, it had
dropped nearly 30 points.

Stephen, a 46-year-old Clinton, New Jersey, resident and
professor of business at Rutgers University, was first diagnosed with high cholesterol in October 1996. Back then, his
HDL was 36, and his LDL was 174. At his next checkup in
May 1999, his total cholesterol was 213, with an HDL of 49
and an LDL of 108. He and his doctor were delighted.

At that time, Stephen was playing basketball with friends
on a weekly basis. He was also swimming about once a
week. He gave up basketball about 2 years later and increased his lap swimming workouts—about 45 minutes each
dip—to three times a week, a practice he continues. He also
walks for 30 minutes once or twice a day.

Other than adding the wine, Stephen made few modifica-
tions to his diet. He changed from 1% milk to fat-free milk
and added organic low-fat yogurt to his lunch bag. But he already ate little meat and very few eggs.

"I tend to avoid fried foods, and I am not a big cheese
eater," he adds. "I will continue to drink the wine. That's the
only major change I made."

W I N N I N G   A C T I O N

Enjoy a glass of red wine with dinner. If you're already a wine drinker, you may be doing your heart good. The protective effect of wine has been attributed to antioxidants in the skin and seeds of red grapes. Some scientists believe that these antioxidants, called flavonoids, reduce the risk of coronary heart disease by inhibiting production of LDL, by boosting production of HDL, and by preventing blood clotting. A 4-ounce glass of wine is equivalent to one serving. Men might benefit from one to two servings per day; women should limit themselves to one serving.

Of course, if you're a teetotaler, you shouldn't start drinking just to get the benefits of the flavonoids. You can get the same heart-healthy nutrients from nonalcoholic purple grape juice.

+++

HE FOUND OUT SOMETHING HORSES HAVE KNOWN ALL ALONG

William Israel was not a great fan of oatmeal. But he was willing to try anything to get his cholesterol down.

"I got a letter from my doctor on May 13, 1998," says William, 83, who lives in Sun Lakes, Arizona. "It said that my cholesterol was 254 and told me what foods to avoid."

William cut out red meats. He added more fruits and vegetables to his diet. And after his wife, Beverly, read an article about the benefits of oatmeal, he added a bowl of the grain, flavored with brown sugar and raisins, to his breakfast regimen. He also started eating oatmeal muffins.

Just over a month later, his cholesterol had dropped to 200. By August 1998, it was 171, the level at which it remains. His HDL is 37, his LDL is 106, and his triglycerides are 140.

William also lost weight. At 5 feet 11 inches, he had weighed 191 pounds. Now he's down to 181.

And in the bargain, the Sun Lakes chapter of the American Heart Association received a check from Quaker for $1,000. How'd that come about?

"My wife said to me, 'Why don't you write a letter to Quaker Oats?'" William says. As a result of his letter describing the benefits of an oatmeal-rich diet, Sun Lakes was recognized by the Quaker Oats Smart Heart Challenge as one of 10 communities in the United States that focus on healthy hearts. The AHA chapter received the check, and William had his picture taken to decorate the Quaker Oats box. (A final decision on whether his picture will ever appear on the box is still pending.)

William was always an active person. A native of Buffalo, New York, he was the president of a furniture company and was active in fund-raising activities in his hometown. After retiring to Sun Lakes 10 years ago, he became a volunteer for the United Way and got involved in the Sun Lakes Jewish Men's Club and the Jewish Congregation. He is also a volunteer for the hospital in a retirement community and is currently raising money to help Neighbors Who Care (a nonprofit organization that helps out wherever needed) buy a van. He also works part-time for Ed Robson, who developed Sun Lakes.

"I feel good, and I am completely involved," William says. In 2000, he underwent hip replacement surgery and treatment for eye cancer. Ten months later, he was back to walking a half-hour to an hour daily. He says he feels great.

"I want to enjoy life," he says. "I want to enjoy my family. Occasionally, I have a couple of eggs and a strip of bacon for breakfast. But I always go back to my oatmeal."

WINNING ACTION

Eat oatmeal. Oats (as well as barley) are great sources of beta glucan, a type of soluble fiber that helps lower total and LDL cholesterol. And oats are not just for breakfast. As William Israel discovered, they make good muffins. They can also be used in pancakes, breads, cookies, meat loaf, and lots of other dishes. Research has shown that 3 grams daily of oat soluble fiber will help lower cholesterol in 30 days. This is the amount in ¾ cup of uncooked rolled oats, which makes 1½ cups of cooked oatmeal.

++

SOY FOODS HELP KEEP
HER CHOLESTEROL IN CHECK

When Shelly Solomon cooks for her family, she doesn't reveal all the ingredients until the meal is over.

That's because Shelly has a tendency to sneak tofu into her recipes. She puts it in her chili, crumbles it into her Egg Beaters omelettes, and uses it in her casseroles. "With tofu, you can stick it in anything, and it absorbs the flavor of whatever you're making," she says. "My husband didn't even know it was in the chili."

Shelly, who's 57 and owns an advertising agency in Chesterfield, Missouri, has long known that what you eat can make a big difference in your health. Twenty-five years ago, she went to a nurse for help in overcoming premenstrual syndrome and learned that avoiding salt, fried foods, alcohol, sugar, and red meat could help reduce the symptoms. "I've always been in the business world, and it's not very professional to be up and down emotionally," she says.

The first time she tried eating tofu was 15 years ago, and it was an experiment that failed miserably, even for Shelly. "It was really mushy, and I tried to do a few things with it. But my family just said, 'This is awful,'" she recalls. "Even I thought, If I'm going to die 10 years earlier, then I'm going to die 10 years earlier."

Still, the news reports about the health benefits of soy kept coming, and a couple of years ago, Shelly decided to give soy another try. A few of her relatives had had breast cancer and colon cancer, and Shelly was hoping soy would lower her own risk. "I wasn't really thinking about cholesterol lowering," she says. "I was just thinking that hopefully I'm not going to get cancer."

But the more immediate effect was on her cholesterol, which had hit a high of 280 in 1996. Even after taking Pravachol, giving up what little fat was left in her diet, such as dark chicken meat, and walking and doing yoga regularly, her cholesterol was still at 220. Eating soy every day for about a year and continuing to take Pravachol brought it down to a healthy 160.

These days, Shelly eats soy every other day, be it soy veggie burgers, soy bacon, or chunks of tofu in a salad. "My boys think I'm nuts," she says. "They're grown and gone, but when they come home, they never know what I'm going to give them. And I never tell them what they're eating until after it's gone. Morningstar Farms makes these veggie 'chicken nuggets' and 'Buffalo wings,' and my family cannot tell the difference. I pride myself on tricking my family."

WINNING ACTION

Try eating more soy foods. There's lots to choose from, including tofu, tempeh, and soy-based meat alternatives. Although studies on the benefits of soy in the prevention of breast cancer are mixed, experts believe that soy foods help lower cholesterol and reduce the risk for heart disease. In fact, the FDA allows food manufacturers of soy protein products to say so on their product labels.

++

HE KNOWS THE FACTS ABOUT FLAX

In 1996, when Ted Bohdan's cholesterol went over 240 for the first time, his doctor didn't seem all that concerned. The only advice Ted received was to stop eating eggs.

A year later, his cholesterol hadn't budged. Ted decided to take matters into his own hands. He paid a visit to his local health food store, where he picked up a bottle of flaxseed. "I had gotten all this literature about medication and other treatments for high cholesterol, but one article caught my attention," says Ted, an 84-year-old retired sales manager from Flushing, New York. "It said that flaxseed could help lower cholesterol. So I decided to try it. And it really worked."

At the time, Ted was already being treated for high blood pressure. It had been diagnosed in 1997, shortly after his wife passed away. "Because of my high blood pressure, I figured I should do what I could to control my cholesterol, too," he says.

Following his doctor's advice, he gave up the two eggs he had routinely eaten for breakfast. He also eliminated butter and ice cream, both of which are high in fat and cholesterol. And he began taking 2 tablespoons of ground flaxseed a day.

Ted mixes the flaxseed into instant oatmeal, which has replaced his morning eggs. He says that the seed—a product of the same plant that produces fiber for spinning into linen—blends right in, because it tastes so much like oatmeal itself.

Within 6 months of adding flaxseed to his diet, Ted saw his cholesterol drop from a high of 260 to around 200. The good news convinced him to reveal to his doctor what he was doing. His doctor approved, because the flaxseed was obviously working.

At his physical exam in 2000, his LDL remained at a borderline 140, but his HDL was an impressive 63. His triglycerides stood at 101, well within the normal range. "I feel really good," Ted says.

So good, in fact, that even surgery and a 5-day hospital

stay couldn't get him down. In September 2000, after taking large doses of aspirin for a torn ligament, he had to undergo surgery for an intestinal ulcer. Four months later, he showed an 80 percent recovery, which absolutely amazed his doctors. "They couldn't believe I have all this energy," he says. "I'm convinced it's because I eat well and keep my cholesterol low."

WINNING ACTION

Supplement your diet with flaxseed. Flaxseed is a top source of cholesterol-lowering soluble fiber and of alpha-linolenic acid, a polyunsaturated fat similar to the heart-healthy omega-3 fatty acids in fish. Adding it to your diet may help (although you should consult your doctor if you're taking medication or if you have a bowel obstruction). Try mixing it with oatmeal, as Ted did. Oats are another great source of soluble fiber. If you take flaxseed alone, take it with at least 8 ounces of water. Always buy ground flaxseed; your body won't digest whole seeds.

+++

HE SAID CHEERS TO GIVING UP BEER

David Tonkin liked an occasional beer in the evenings, drank a very occasional gin and tonic, and would order a few brews if he went out to dinner on weekends. But when his triglycerides topped out at 1,100 in July 2000, he swore off all alcohol and managed to bring his cholesterol as well as his triglycerides to more respectable figures.

David, age 35, had been monitoring his cholesterol since 1992, when it started hovering in the mid-200s. His mother has a history of elevated cholesterol levels, and David wants to avoid heart disease. But he wasn't always vigilant about what he ate, even though his diet consisted of pasta and chicken and an occasional pizza or takeout Chinese. "If I got a poor reading, I would watch my diet for about 6 weeks and stay away from saturated fats like red meat and butter," he says. "But then I'd lose interest."

His interest was piqued when he went to see a nutritionist the day after he attended two Fourth of July parties. His triglycerides normally hovered around 400; on this occasion, they had soared to 1,100. "I was so disgusted that I didn't even write down the numbers," says David, a central Massachusetts resident who has kept track of each reading for nearly a decade. "It scared the hell out of me, and I just made the decision not to waver again."

Exercise was not the issue, since David was lifting weights regularly. But he did change his diet. He started eating more fruits, vegetables, and fish and switched from white rice to brown rice, from white pasta to the whole wheat variety. He also started taking a 1,000-milligram flaxseed capsule every day and sprinkling ground flaxseed on his cereal every morning.

And at the suggestion of his nutritionist, he immediately gave up the beers. "I used to drink four to six beers a week, usually on the weekends or at night after dinner," he says. "Now I'll have maybe two nonalcoholic beers during the week, just if I want that taste." Instead, he drinks a lot of water and diet sodas.

Giving up alcohol paid off quickly. Less than 2 months after his triglycerides were at 1,100, they were down to 173, well below what they had ever been. His total cholesterol, which had hit a high of 296 in September 1998, had dropped to 218.

"It's just a matter of watching what you put in your mouth and not taking a day off," David says.

W I N N I N G   A C T I O N

If you imbibe, count your glasses. A little alcohol can do your heart good. Studies have shown that moderate consumption—one drink per day for women, two drinks for men—may actually raise HDL, the good cholesterol, and help prevent blood from clotting. But imbibe too much, and alcohol can have the opposite effect, elevating triglycerides and blood pressure, which are both risk factors for heart disease. For some people, even small amounts of alcohol can be harmful.

The best advice? If you don't drink, don't start. If you do drink, be sure to keep it moderate. And if you suspect that alcohol may be having an adverse effect on your cholesterol, talk with your doctor.

+++

SITTING QUIETLY BRINGS HIM RESULTS TO SHOUT ABOUT

After having a heart attack in 1989, Don Vaupel was told to get his affairs in order. His doctors gave him just 4 months to live.

Three months later, Don was enrolled in Dr. Dean Ornish's Program for Reversing Heart Disease—and inspiring the rest of his family to take charge of their heart health. "My mother's total cholesterol was over 400," says Don, an Oakland, California, resident. "She and others in my family saw that I had survived and beaten the odds, so they followed my example." That example involved a combination of nutritious eating, exercise, meditation, visualization, and light yoga.

Even before his heart attack, Don had made changes in his diet that would ultimately affect his heart health. Decades before, he had given up beef and pork after touring a meat-packing plant. And he had sworn off eggs because of an allergy. Still, his eating habits left a lot to be desired. "One of my favorite snacks was french fries and mayonnaise," he confesses.

That combination wouldn't have a place in the Ornish program, which advocates a plant-based eating plan that limits fat intake to just 10 percent of calories. With a guideline like that, you might think that eating in restaurants is out of the question. But Don manages it easily. "Believe it or not, one of the best places to get a vegetarian meal is in a steakhouse," he says. "They have great potatoes, salad bars, and vegetable selections. You can load up on side dishes and do well."

While cutting back on dietary fat undoubtedly had a major impact on his heart health, Don feels he may have gotten even greater benefit from the meditation component of the Ornish program. He started by setting aside just 5 minutes twice a day—at the same times each day—to "relax and do nothing." It enabled him to put his life in perspective—and to change it for the better.

"After my first heart attack, I returned to my job as a college administrator, and over the next 2 years, I had several mini cardiac events," Don says. "All of them happened on the job, and each one brought chest pain, indigestion, sweating, and fatigue.

"People involved with the Ornish program advised me to leave my job, but I was stubborn," he continues. "While meditation was steering me in the right direction and possibly protecting me from another full-blown heart attack, my whole lifestyle was still stress, stress, stress, stress."

Finally, while lying in the hospital for the fifth time, Don could no longer ignore the constant assault on his health. He signed his disability papers and took early retirement. "I came to understand the importance of stress management," he says. "It makes everything easier: eating healthfully, dealing with people, dealing with life itself."

These days, Don has plenty of time for meditation—and he takes advantage of it. He fits in two 1-hour sessions a day.

"That time is important to me," he says. "Meditating gives me clarity and helps me make better decisions."

Don continues to follow the rest of the Ornish program as well. At age 62, he hasn't had any more chest pain, and he feels better than he has in years. His total cholesterol has dropped from 232 at the time of his first heart attack to an impressive 126.

Even though he's retired, Don occasionally serves as a health consultant, helping others to follow the Ornish program—especially the meditation component. "People have the most trouble learning how to sit or lie quietly and meditate," he says. But he keeps encouraging them until they start noticing the benefits. "People treat themselves worse than they treat their cars," he says. "Quiet time lets your body slow down, assess itself, and heal. Your body will tell you everything if only you listen to it."

WINNING ACTION

Tune in to yourself, turn down your cholesterol. Excess stress often contributes to overeating and other behaviors that can negatively affect your cholesterol level and your overall health. Daily meditation—first thing in the morning, over your lunch hour, or right before bed—will help you relax and reconnect with yourself. You can use that time to assess various lifestyle choices that you've made during the day—what to have for breakfast, whether to exercise—and make adjustments. You'll feel that you have more control over your health, and that can make a big difference in your cholesterol level.

++

HE PUT WORK IN ITS PLACE
AND IMPROVED HIS HEALTH

"When I graduated from law school, I promised that I would never turn into a workaholic like other successful lawyers whom I admired," says Ron Major, a 54-year-old Cincinnati resident.

Unfortunately, a workaholic is exactly what Ron became. By the mid-1990s, 20 years into his law career, Ron found his physical and emotional health deteriorating. "I had exercised regularly at the Cincinnati Athletic Club, swimming a mile every morning and using the Nautilus machines three times a week," he says. "I quit the Athletic Club because I couldn't afford the time for working out.

"My diet consisted of five cups of coffee for breakfast and crackers and a diet soft drink at my desk for lunch. Dinner was whatever passed through my car window at the fast-food restaurant on the way home," says Ron. "The number of days spent in the office went from 5 to 6 and eventually to 7."

Thirty pounds overweight, with a total cholesterol level over 250, Ron had a heart attack just after completing a trial in July 1997. His wife, Karen, a registered nurse, helped rush him to an emergency room, where he received an emergency angioplasty.

"I was one of the lucky few who survive the first heart attack," says Ron, "and I was determined that I was going to do everything in my power to take advantage of this gift from God."

While still in the hospital, Ron began a cardiac rehabilitation program of controlled exercise. "I met other cardiac patients, including lawyers, judges, and doctors whose lives were remarkably similar to mine," he says.

A personal trainer then helped him develop a three-times-a-week workout of 30 minutes on a treadmill followed by an hour of strength training with free weights. "I also began swimming again," says Ron. "While I initially could swim only six to eight laps without gasping for air, I've now worked back up to a mile."

Ron's diet underwent similar improvement. "I have a protein shake and bagel for breakfast, a grilled chicken sandwich or other protein source plus fruit for lunch, and a balanced meal for dinner," he says. One year after his heart attack, his weight was down to 205 (a 20-pound drop for the 5-foot-10 attorney), and his total cholesterol was down to 157.

In addition to taking yoga for relaxation, Ron says that he's reduced his work hours and even leaves the office early once a week to walk with Karen in the nearby parks. Says Ron, "There's nothing like a face-to-face meeting with your own mortality to remind you of what is truly important in your life."

WINNING ACTION

Keep your job out of the rest of your life. Working long hours or on weekends will earn you extra money, but you might end up spending it all on the hospital bill. If you want to enjoy—or more important, survive—the decades after you retire, put the work aside and take the time to eat right and exercise. If your boss questions your commitment, explain that you want to be in tip-top shape so that you can do your best for years to come—and that's no lie!

++

RELAXATION REINED IN
HER CHOLESTEROL

As a speech communication professor, Joanna Pucel teaches others how to relax before presentations. She could have used some lessons in relaxation herself. It took triple bypass surgery to convince her to put the brakes on her fast-paced lifestyle and build in some downtime.

Not that stress was the only factor putting Joanna at risk for high cholesterol and heart disease. "My family history is horrendous," says the 54-year-old St. Cloud, Minnesota, resident. "My mother's side of the family had 12 siblings, and most of my aunts and uncles died from heart attacks before they turned 30."

Joanna was just 37 when she had her triple bypass. She went to the doctor because she had been experiencing difficulty breathing. A blood test found her total cholesterol to be a frighteningly high 295, with an LDL of 238, HDL of 48, and triglycerides of 46. "I was shocked," she recalls. "I had a relatively healthy diet, and I played tennis regularly. I wasn't overweight, and I never smoked."

Even though she seemed to be doing everything right, her arteries suggested otherwise. During an angiogram (a test of the heart's blood vessels), her doctors detected a blocked coronary artery; they concluded that she was about a week away from a heart attack. In surgery, they made a more disturbing discovery: Joanna had had a silent heart attack about 30 years earlier, and part of her heart was no longer functioning.

That news left Joanna more determined than ever to rein in her cholesterol. She made further adjustments in her diet, switching from cooking oils to sprays and eating even more fruit and bran. She invested in a treadmill, which she used on days when she didn't play tennis. Three years after her surgery, with help from Colestid and later Mevacor, her total cholesterol finally dipped below 200. Her HDL rose to 64, her LDL dropped to 104, and her triglycerides inched up to 75.

Unfortunately, they didn't stay there. At age 48, Joanna had a hysterectomy that left her without the protective effects of estrogen. Her cholesterol rose to 290. "I kept asking myself, Why can't I get it down?" Joanna says. "I felt that I was missing something."

Through her own research, she uncovered a suspected connection between stress and cholesterol. She knew that she had found her culprit. Between her workload—she's on the faculty of St. Cloud State University in Minnesota—and her many civic activities, she often felt overwhelmed.

To rein in her stress, Joanna started setting priorities. She stopped teaching summer school, turned down requests to hold offices for civic groups, and even put less pressure on herself to exercise. "I'm constantly asking myself, What must I get done, and what can wait?" she says. "Some things just get put off until the next day."

Joanna has found other ways to destress, too. She goes out to lunch with her tennis buddies and has learned crafts such as basket making. Every weekend, she spends at least an hour puttering around her greenhouse. And every night, she sets aside at least 15 minutes to soak in a hot bath scented with her favorite bubblebath. "If my husband and I get home after midnight, he'll go to bed, and I'll still take my hot bath," she says. "Nothing is worse than going to bed tense, and a bath literally washes away all the tension. It has become a ritual for me."

Judging by her latest cholesterol test, Joanna's stress reduction efforts have been a success. Her total cholesterol is down to 209, with an LDL of 107, HDL of 91, and triglycerides of 53. While she'd like to get her total cholesterol level even lower, she'll be content if it stays in the neighborhood of 200.

Joanna is even more pleased with her new stress-free attitude toward life. "Before, when I had a lot of work to do, I would have stayed up until midnight or 1 o'clock in the morning to finish it," she says. "Now, no matter what's on my plate, I make sure to schedule relaxation into my day. It helps me avoid the late nights by keeping me focused on what's really important."

WINNING ACTION

Schedule relaxation breaks into your day. A little stress can be a good thing. But too much for too long can raise your risk of a heart attack—especially if you also have high cholesterol as a risk factor. According to the National Heart, Lung, and Blood Institute of the National Institutes of Health, stress can contribute to unhealthy eating habits that make high cholesterol even worse. So no matter how busy you are, make time to unwind. Even 10 minutes of walking or deep breathing can defuse your body's stress response and protect your heart from harm.

++

RAIN OR SHINE, NATURE BOOSTS HIS SPIRIT

Clay Leath was a meat-and-potatoes man. He devoured sweets, especially chocolate, and rarely exercised.

Today, an angioplasty later, the chocolate and potatoes are gone, and the meat is lean only. And two walks a day, every day, are part of his routine.

"I love being outdoors," says Clay. "It is something I look forward to: getting outside, walking, and thinking about everything I need to think about."

Clay, a 57-year-old Richardson, Texas, resident, is retired from the military and is a financial systems support manager for the Dallas office of the American Heart Association (AHA). "I sit in an office all day, and I only get outside for my walks," he says. "They give me time to stop and smell the roses. The diet that I am on is good, but I certainly couldn't do it without the walking."

He walks 2 miles every morning. In the evening, he, his wife, Asako, and their dog, Momo, walk another 2 miles. Rain, shine, and even in the Texas heat.

In February 1999, Clay started having pain in his left arm and chest as well as nausea. A stress test confirmed that at least one artery leading to his heart was blocked. His total cholesterol was 246.

As it turned out, there was only one blockage, and the angioplasty cleared it up. But the procedure was not a pleasant experience, according to Clay. And when he read that up to 25 percent of people who undergo angioplasty need to have it done again, he was determined to do everything he could to get his cholesterol down. He also wanted to slim down; at 5 feet 9, he weighed 246 pounds.

His doctor suggested that he follow eating guidelines recommended by the AHA. "I was thinking that I would never be able to eat anything good again," Clay says. But he purchased an AHA cookbook, and his wife began preparing dishes—low-fat, low-sugar, and low-salt—from it. "They are very good," Clay says.

Between his dietary changes and his walks, Clay lowered his cholesterol to 161. He also lost 41 pounds, but regained some of it during the 2000 holiday season. Now he's holding steady at 215.

Besides lower cholesterol and a trimmer physique, Clay has noticed other improvements in his health. "My energy has really gone up tremendously," he says. "I have a 19-month-old granddaughter, and my goal is to see her graduate from college. I am proud of what I have done. And proud that I could do it without medicine."

WINNING ACTION

Get outside. Study after study has shown that regular physical activity is associated with a reduced risk of cardiovascular disease for people of any age. As creatures of nature, we sometimes long to be free of wood and concrete. Our spirits soar when we are outside, and so does our

*determination to do the right thing, such as stick to a diet.
Whether your passion is walking, cycling, playing sports, or
jogging, the time you spend outdoors can have a direct
effect on your cholesterol, weight, and overall health.*

++

HE CUT BACK ON WORK HOURS AND
FOUND TIME FOR HIS HEALTH

As the oldest son of a dairy farmer, Larry Stall had a very active lifestyle in his youth. But in his grown-up job as a software engineer in Milton, Wisconsin, physical activity had all
but vanished. "I sat in front of a computer all day at work,
then went home and did the same," he says. "I was becoming
a very successful programmer while my health was going
down the tubes."

That all changed in May 1998, when Larry, then 46, had a
heart attack. Suddenly, his cholesterol, which had topped 300
for the past 10 years, took on great importance. He dropped
his 28-year, two-pack-a-day cigarette habit in the hospital
and started taking Zocor (later switching to Lipitor) under
doctor's orders. But he still felt shaky, broken up, unsure how
to go on.

To get back to normal, he tried to immerse himself in his
job. He found it impossible. "I couldn't shake the memory
that while I was having my attack—and wasn't sure whether
I would live or die—I realized that my job was pretty unim-
portant compared with my family and my life," says Larry.
"As I began to recognize the stress I had been under, I even
resented my job."

Larry decided to cut back on overtime at work and loung-
ing time at home, instead devoting that time to exercise. "I
went from sporadic activity to a regular schedule at a health
club, where I work out at least three times a week for 2 hours
each time," he says. "I also exchanged sedentary hobbies like

photography and computers for more active ones like biking, hiking, and running. I probably exercise at least 12 hours a week now."

He also made numerous diet changes to limit calories from fat to less than 30 percent of his daily intake. "I've eliminated butter and standard pastries," he says. "I've reduced the amount of red meat and increased the percentage of fish, seafood, and poultry."

Within 4 months of his heart attack and the subsequent diet and exercise changes, Larry reduced his total cholesterol from a high of 316 in March 1998 to 161. Along the way, his triglyceride level dropped from 208 to 112 and his LDL level from 230 all the way to 80. Another year's worth of work doubled his HDL, from 30 to 59.

In addition to rosier cholesterol numbers, his weight has fallen from 210 to 168. "I have more energy and stamina and feel better than I have in about 20 years!" says Larry, who's now 49. "I only wish I had known how good I could feel—or how bad I was actually feeling—all those years that I ignored my health."

WINNING ACTION

Drop the overtime to lose stress. The relationship between heart disease and stress isn't exactly clear, but people under stress tend to overeat, smoke more, and exercise less—all of which tend to increase cholesterol. Working overtime, especially on projects that make or break the company, is a sure way to boost stress levels beyond what's tolerable. If your health suffers, your work will suffer as well, so make sure that your boss understands the connection. Either punch out at 5:00 P.M. and head for a home-cooked meal rather than a vending machine dinner or ask the company to bring other employees in to work with you.

++

PRAYER GAVE HIM THE STRENGTH TO FIGHT HEART DISEASE

Harry Deen was a self-described workaholic, the kind of man who literally had a heart attack one day and went to work the next. But when heart disease threatened his life and Harry sank into depression, it was the slow, calming effects of prayer that put him on the path to recovery.

For 18 years, Harry owned a 300-seat steakhouse on the beaches of Panama City, Florida. He worked 12 to 14 hours a day, 7 days a week, cutting as many as 300 steaks a day and doing all his own cooking. When he had his first heart attack at age 42, he went home, only to return to work the next day. "It was the only time I ever left the steakhouse early and went home early," recalls Harry, now 61. "I didn't even go to the doctor."

But in 1992, at the age of 52, Harry had a massive heart attack and underwent bypass surgery. He wound up staying in the hospital's intensive care unit for a month after his sutures broke and he contracted a staph infection in his chest. His cholesterol at the time was at a high of 215.

When he finally left the hospital, Harry had enormous bills. He tried to work but no longer had the strength. His business faltered and closed. Although he had insurance, it wasn't nearly enough to pay off a quarter-million dollars in medical bills. He resorted to credit cards and eventually lost his home and car.

To make matters worse, in 1994, doctors discovered a new blockage near his heart and a failed bypass graft to the right coronary artery from the previous surgery. Harry fell into a deep depression. "I was just waiting to die," he says. "I kept thinking, Tomorrow I won't wake up."

For solace, he began taking short walks to isolated areas of a state park on the beach. Harry loved nature because it gave him peace and tranquility. In late afternoon, when most visitors had left the park, Harry would wade into the water of the lagoon or the Gulf of Mexico, float on his back, and pray while staring at the sky.

His early conversations with God were angry ones. "When I was floating, I'd say to God, 'You had me, so why did you send me back to this hell?'" he says.

With each visit to the park, however, Harry walked farther and farther, until after 6 months, he was able to complete the entire 3-mile loop. "It got to where I wasn't feeling the pain anymore," he says. "I realized, I'm not dying, my life is not over."

In 1997, after undergoing an angioplasty and a stent implant, Henry became more proactive in his battle against heart disease. He joined the American Heart Association, entered a cardiac rehabilitation program, and established a heart support group. He read books on health and heart disease by Dean Ornish, M.D., Kenneth Cooper, M.D., and Andrew Weil, M.D. He started doing yoga, cut back on red meat, and ate more fish.

In 1998, after months of monitoring his diet and exercising regularly, Harry saw his total cholesterol hit an all-time low of 99. It has remained under 110 ever since.

While his cholesterol is better than ever, Harry still has a few health problems to contend with. He has arterial blockages in places that can't be treated with angioplasty. His left leg is affected by peripheral artery disease, which he's able to control with walking. And although he quit his 30-year cigarette habit, he has emphysema.

Harry no longer spends afternoons floating on his back and praying. But he stills talks to God and gives Him credit for guiding him onto the path of recovery. "I'm always thankful to God for pulling me through," says Harry, who was recently named vice president of his local heart association. "Now I've got my life back in control. I can truthfully say, 'Life is good.'"

W I N N I N G   A C T I O N

Look to prayer for the strength to improve. When every-thing seems hopeless, pray to a higher authority for strength. Putting faith in a supreme being relieves stress and helps you focus on other priorities, such as taking steps to make your health better. Prayer can help you stay centered and give you the strength to pursue goals toward greater well-being.

+++

HE EDUCATED HIMSELF ABOUT CHOLESTEROL CONTROL

When Mark McKelvey's cholesterol hit 491, his doctor had one immediate piece of advice.

"He told me to get on Mevacor, a cholesterol-fighting statin drug, right away," says Mark, 44, of Saugus, California. "But I was apprehensive about taking medicine. I am not a drug kind of guy. I am a natural kind of guy."

So Mark, who was about 30 when he was diagnosed with familial hypercholesterolemia, a genetic tendency toward high cholesterol, started reading everything he could find about nondrug alternatives for controlling cholesterol and pre-venting heart disease. Within 8 weeks of putting his newfound knowledge into practice, he had lowered his total cholesterol to 169. His ratio of total cholesterol to HDL also plummeted from a dangerously high 14 to a healthy 3.5.

In the process, Mark managed to lose 17 pounds. At 5 feet 10 inches, he had weighed 185. Now, at 168, "I look good and feel good," he says proudly.

So what did Mark learn in his reading? First, from *Diet for New America* by John Robbins, he discovered the benefits of a vegan diet. "I read the book nonstop in 14 hours," he says. "It blew me away."

He eliminated all animal products, including dairy foods, from his diet. In their place, he chose protein-packed vegetables and soy. (In an experimental mood, he added cheese to his meals a few years later. His cholesterol climbed to 240.) "I kind of missed meat at first, but now I find it disgusting," he says.

Mark also eliminated hydrogenated oils. "Udo Erasmus wrote the bible on fats and oils," he says. "I avoid hydrogenated oils like the plague."

From the writings of Linus Pauling, Ph.D., Mark learned of Abram Hoffer's discovery of the cholesterol-lowering benefits of niacin. Mark began taking daily doses of the B vitamin, along with vitamin C, vitamin E, and the amino acid lysine. All of these supplements were recommended by Dr. Pauling to prevent cholesterol from oxidizing and clogging arteries, Mark says.

All told, Mark spends $10 a day on supplements. But it is well worth it. "I like being alive," he says. "I want my family to grow up with a dad."

And he wants his daughter, 5, who inherited her father's tendency to high cholesterol, to have a healthy life. "She's being raised a vegetarian, and she takes a multivitamin and vitamin C every day," Mark says. "I like to know all I can, so my daughter doesn't have any problems as she grows older."

WINNING ACTION

Read, read, and read some more. The more you know about cholesterol problems, the better able you'll be to help yourself and work with your doctor to get your levels down. And since new studies are constantly uncovering fresh approaches to cholesterol management, keep your research ongoing. Look to health newsletters, books, and the Internet; some Web sites to consider are

www.americanheart.org (the American Heart Associa-
tion), www.webmd.com, and www.prevention.com. But
always discuss the information with your doctor.

++

SHE COUNTED POINTS—AND COUNTED HERSELF HEALTHIER

In the early 1980s, Pamela Thomas's cholesterol was 250, but she didn't care. By 2000, when she turned 44, this Garland, Texas, native cared a lot.

Pamela is a smoker, and her mother once had a mild stroke. She knew that these factors, plus the high cholesterol, put her at risk for heart problems. Not only that, but in June 2000, "My doctor told me to get my cholesterol levels down and to lose weight or he couldn't do anything for me anymore," she says. "I really like my current doctor, and I wanted to become healthier and live a long, productive life."

Pamela joined Weight Watchers on August 5, 2000, weighing in at 207 pounds. "And I'm only 5 feet 4," she says. By her next checkup, just 3 weeks later, she had already lost 6 pounds—an encouraging sign. "So joining Weight Watchers, counting the points, and cutting down on portions, junk food, and soda—I was drinking an average of four a day—really did help," she says. She also learned to eat more fruits and veggies, to have soup to take the edge off her hunger, and to drink at least eight glasses of water per day.

Pamela's husband was behind her efforts all the way. He even started preparing menus from a Weight Watchers book and reading the side panels on foods for nutrition information.

Within a month of joining Weight Watchers, and with a little help from Lipitor, Pamela's cholesterol level dropped to 182. Within 5 months, she had lost 20 pounds. Now she's cutting down on cigarettes, and she has started an exercise program that combines walking and strength training to boost her health even more.

"I am so tickled pink that I have lost weight and inches and in the process gotten much healthier," says Pamela. "Life is too short to be overweight and have high cholesterol. Just make a decision to lose weight, talk with your doctor, and get going. Everyone deserves a new wardrobe."

WINNING ACTION

Don't go it alone. Join a weight-loss group to learn the basics of healthy living and to share experiences with other people who are overcoming their weight and cholesterol problems. And don't think you have to seek out a national organization to get the benefits—call your local fitness center or hospital and ask if a weight-loss group meets there. A group of any size will teach you healthy habits, and you'll be reinforced and encouraged by the other members.

++

HE WENT BACK TO SCHOOL TO EARN A DEGREE IN GOOD HEALTH

At age 71, Earl Brensinger is fighting history. His father died of a heart attack, his brother underwent open-heart surgery, and Earl himself had surgery to clean out an artery in his neck that was 95 percent blocked.

Before the surgery, Earl's total cholesterol level was 240. This, on top of two ministrokes in 1998 and the type 2 diabetes that came on in 1992, prompted his doctor to invite Earl to participate in a new study at Lehigh Valley Hospital in Allentown, Pennsylvania, called LOVAR (Lowering of Vascular Atherosclerotic Risk).

This 5-year study, funded by the Dorothy Rider Pool Health Care Trust, is trying to determine whether an integrated program of lifestyle behavior modification and stress management can help high-risk patients alter their risk factors and improve their quality of life. Earl attends classes at the hospital two or three times a week for 2 to 3 hours at a time, learning about topics like cholesterol, stroke, heart attack, stress management, exercise, and diet and nutrition. "All of the instructors are nurses, dietitians, and health educators, and they know their subjects inside and out," he says. "If you couldn't learn from them, you couldn't learn from anybody."

"I've learned a lot that I wouldn't have known about if I wasn't in the program," says Earl, who lives in Emmaus, Pennsylvania. "It's helped to control my blood sugar, which is especially important since I'm diabetic."

He's also learned how to control his portion sizes and how to choose food that better fits his needs. "They allow you only 6 ounces of red meat a week, which is only a medium-sized hamburger," he says. "And just because you can't eat red meat doesn't mean you can go out and eat a pound of fish. It doesn't work that way."

Unlike during his work years, Earl now walks 2½ to 3 miles a day, no matter what the conditions outside are. "If the weather is bad, I go over to the mall and do a few laps," he says. If he can't get out and walk for some reason, he does aerobics instead.

One year after undergoing surgery to reduce his odds of having a major stroke, Earl has reduced his total cholesterol to 148, and his LDL level stands at an impressive 84.

All this interest in health care is a big change from the time Earl spent as the town's police chief. "I was behind the desk 7 out of 8 hours of the day, so I got very little exercise," he says. "I wish I had had a program like this then. It would have helped a lot."

W I N N I N G   A C T I O N

Find a hospital-sponsored cholesterol program. Don't wait until you're ready to have surgery to learn about cholesterol-reducing programs in your vicinity. Ask your physician or nutritionist for information about programs or studies that you can participate in now. Not every town or city has one, but if you keep asking your doctor and showing interest in the topic, perhaps the hospital will create a program to meet the needs of the community.

+++

STAY ON TRACK
FOR SUCCESS

✦ ✦ ✦

SHE TURNED HER MIDLIFE CRISIS
INTO AN OPPORTUNITY

As a medical technologist and laboratory manager, Carole DeMartino was able to check her health stats anytime she felt like it. But that doesn't mean they were always good. "My cholesterol was high, my triglycerides were high, my lipid profile was terrible," she says. "I knew what the numbers were, but they didn't seem enough to stop me."

That is, not until one day in July 1994, when she happened to step on a scale at work and found that she weighed 265 pounds. Since she's only 5 feet 4, this—on top of high blood pressure, borderline diabetes, and a total cholesterol level of 285—finally drove her into action.

For the next 2 weeks, she limited her diet to fruit, vegetables, and fish, eating as much as she wanted to stave off hunger. Soon, she added whole grains, beans, and nuts to establish a more balanced approach to her meals. She had tried fad diets all her life, but now that she had created a food plan of her own, she found it much easier to stick to.

Even though the diet was a big change for her, "exercise is probably the most important thing," says Carole, who's 57 and lives in Bloomfield, New Jersey. Her first walk, ½ mile around the block, knocked the wind out of her, but she did it again the next day. And the day after that. And she kept at it until she was walking the 2-mile round trip to work each day—and looking for more.

"The more I exercised, the more my body got used to it and became unresponsive," says Carole. "I found that I had to keep varying intensities and exercise routines." She sought out hills for muscle toning and developed a "six-level" walk in which she'd vary the intensity of the walk as it progressed. "I think that makes a huge difference," she says.

Although her new lifestyle had been prompted by weight concerns, her cholesterol benefited from the change of habit as well. "As I was losing weight and exercising, I could see the cholesterol going down," says Carole. "There was a time when my triglycerides were down to 30, and my HDL level was up to 87 or 88. I was the talk of the laboratory."

Two years after Carole took up the fruit and hit the road, she had lost 120 pounds and brought her total cholesterol level down to 180—a figure that she's maintained to this day. "It's almost religious to me now," she says. "I'm very fervent about it. When I go on vacation, I carry my weights with me. Instead of going to lunch, I take an hour's walk each day, and if I don't, I feel deprived. I think I'm addicted to exercise now."

WINNING ACTION

Turn a crisis into an opportunity for change. Don't assume that just because you've reached middle age, your body is going to fall apart. Your body is only as bad—or as good—as what you put into it and what you do to it. If you treat it well, giving it low-fat, healthy fuel to run on and exercising it well, it will serve you for decades to come.

+++

AFTER HIS HEART ATTACKED, HE STRUCK BACK

You think your job is stressful? Talk to Bill Pantle, a 30-year veteran of the air force and a 12½-year survivor of open-heart surgery. Bill started his air force career as a B-52 navigator-bombardier, went on to fly as a weapons systems officer, and then stepped into military intelligence.

As his career climbed, so did his total cholesterol. It peaked at 278 in 1981, while Bill was assigned as the director of operational intelligence. His diet at the time didn't help much. "I ate lots of red meat and dairy," he recalls. In the morning, "my wife would hand me a sandwich consisting of three scrambled eggs and several slices of bacon."

After receiving nutrition counseling, Bill started eating smaller and leaner cuts of red meat, lots of broiled chicken, and steamed vegetables. In the morning, he sat down to oatmeal instead of bacon and eggs. By the time he retired in the fall of 1988, his total cholesterol level had fallen to 235.

Unfortunately, that improvement wasn't enough to undo the years of stress and smoking (he quit in 1973) he had put his body through. On New Year's Day 1989, Bill, who had been admitted to the hospital for cardiac symptoms and some changes in his EKG, had a heart attack.

But he didn't let it set him back for long. "Just like possession is nine-tenths of the law, attitude is nine-tenths of recovery," says Bill. "Lying in the hospital and not knowing what was ahead of me, I started looking at the things I could do as opposed to what I would not be capable of doing."

Following open-heart surgery, his doctors told him to walk

twice a day, going longer and faster each time. Since it was midwinter, Bill headed over to the firehouse to get his track time in. "Do you have any idea how many different patterns you can walk around four parked fire trucks?" he asks. He also started swimming, and within 8 weeks of his surgery, he could cover a mile in the pool.

Bill got even more serious about the diet he had started in the air force, inventing recipes for omelettes with egg substitute and for muffins and pancakes with oat bran. "You eat one of those muffins in the morning, and at 2:00 in the afternoon, you can feel your liver sucking cholesterol out of your bloodstream," he says.

Today, at age 65, Bill sports a healthy cholesterol level of 161. He's running his own consulting firm in Rome, New York, and still swimming three mornings a week, in addition to backpacking and canoeing. His diet is as healthy as ever. He's also president of his local chapter of Mended Hearts, a national support group for heart patients and their families.

"You have to make a commitment, change your attitude, and change your lifestyle," says Bill. "You know what your risk factors are. If there's heart disease in your family, you can work on those risk factors. You owe it to yourself and your family to do it."

WINNING ACTION

Act on what you can and ignore what you can't. You can't shake your genetic history, and it's unlikely that you can change jobs at will, but that doesn't mean you're stuck with high cholesterol. Many risk factors, such as smoking, diets high in cholesterol or saturated fat, and a lack of exercise, are preventable. They can't harm you unless you allow them to, so leave aside the factors you can't change and focus all your energy on eliminating those you can.

++

SHE TOOK CHARGE OF HER LIFE—
AND HER CHOLESTEROL

Andrea Wilkison never had her cholesterol checked before 1998. "Honestly, it hadn't been a concern for me," says the Laramie, Wyoming, resident. "After all, I was only in my late twenties."

As her numbers proved, cholesterol trouble knows no age limit. Her HDL measured a miserly 31, which put her ratio of total cholesterol to HDL at a high-risk 5. "My paternal grandfather died from heart disease, and my father struggled with high cholesterol and blood pressure as well," Andrea explains. "I knew that if I didn't mend my ways, I would be following in their footsteps."

Back when she was a college student, Andrea had maintained a low-fat, mostly vegetarian diet. As her career as a high school teacher flourished and her family grew—she and her husband, Randy, have three children—fast food made up a much larger percentage of her meals. Exercise was nonexistent. At one point, Andrea and Randy even visited a wellness center for advice on how to lose weight, eat better, and incorporate physical activity into their daily routines. But they knew that any changes they made had to come from within themselves.

Because of her family history of high cholesterol and heart disease, Andrea had special incentive to reshape her lifestyle and reduce the risk factors within her control. Number one on her list was to beat stress by exercising rather than eating. "I forced myself to schedule time to work out," she says. "Now, I'd be a nervous wreck if I didn't exercise. It's my stress reliever." She works out for at least 30 minutes 5 days a week. She prefers to walk outside, but if the weather isn't cooperative, she heads to a health club near her home. When she feels herself getting bored at the club, she switches to a new activity to keep herself going.

She has overhauled her diet as well. "My husband and I

don't dine out as often as we used to. We like to have control over what we eat and how it's prepared," Andrea says. "If I do go to a fast food restaurant, I try to order a baked potato or a salad, which is more healthy."

Six months after she started making healthy changes in her diet and lifestyle, Andrea's HDL had risen to an impressive 43, and her ratio had fallen to a much healthier 4. She also made some headway in slimming down, dropping from 186 to 168 (she's 5 feet 4). That's about a third of her goal, but that's okay. "I want to lose the rest of the weight," says Andrea, who's now 33. "But I'm happy just to know that I can have a positive impact on my cholesterol and my health by eating well and exercising almost every day."

WINNING ACTION

Remember: You're in control. You decide whether or not to exercise. You decide whether to eat a burger and fries at a fast food joint or a skinless chicken breast and a salad at home. You decide whether to remain stressed or release your frustrations by working out. Use that power to your advantage by making good eating and exercise choices throughout each day, and you're sure to keep your cholesterol in check!

++

PATIENCE IS . . . A LOWER CHOLESTEROL READING

By all accounts, John O'Keefe is a lucky man. He learned he had dangerously high cholesterol—in the neighborhood of 330—*before* he had a heart attack or required bypass surgery. Getting it under control has taken more than a decade. But

John's patience and persistence have paid off handsomely: His cholesterol has dropped more than 130 points.

With a family history of cholesterol trouble, John wasn't entirely surprised when a routine physical in October 1990 revealed that he, too, had high cholesterol. What astounded him was just how high the number was. "I knew right away that I had to make some changes in my lifestyle," he says.

After he convinced his wife to join him in his efforts, the couple cut out the burgers, cheese steaks, and french fries that had become standard fare two or three times a week. Instead, they ate lots of pasta, fish, and chicken. "Now I get about 2,000 calories per day," says John. "I have no idea how many calories I was consuming before, but I'm sure it was a lot more."

For exercise, John—a runner in his high school days—decided to lace up his running shoes once again. "I thought it would be the easiest activity to pick up," he says. Sure enough, within 3 months, he had regained his old stamina and was covering up to 20 miles a week around his Medford Lakes, New Jersey, home.

John remained faithful to his diet and exercise plans for years. Ever so slowly, his cholesterol crept downward. But by the late 1990s, it plateaued at 220—and neither he nor his doctor was happy. "I couldn't believe it. I ate right, I ran regularly, and still my cholesterol was too high," he says. "I realized that my family was going to be tough to beat."

But John, age 55, has persevered. By sticking with his diet and exercise plans, now in combination with Zocor, he managed to lower his cholesterol to 193 by 2000. "I've not had red meat for more than a decade," he says. "I still run a couple of times a week and follow a low-fat diet, as does my wife. Both of us have benefited from a healthier lifestyle. I know I feel great!"

WINNING ACTION

*Keep your expectations realistic. Lowering your choles-
terol can take a while, and you can't really predict how
effective each step you take is going to be. All you can do
is make the changes, remain consistent in your new behaviors, and see what results. For example, if giving up red
meat doesn't give you good numbers right away, you can
always do more later. The important thing is that you make
the effort and start seeing your cholesterol fall!*

++

A HEALTHY ATTITUDE MAKES
A 130-POINT DIFFERENCE

Kay Bader admits that she had some pretty unhealthy
habits. But she never felt compelled to change until she
found out that her total cholesterol had surpassed 300. The
diagnosis—hypercholesterolemia, or excess cholesterol in
the blood—startled her into action. To her surprise, as she
made her lifestyle healthier, she didn't miss her old habits
one bit.

First on Kay's agenda was snuffing out the cigarette habit
that she had picked up at age 16. "I was up to three packs a
day," recalls the 59-year-old retired draftsperson from La-
Grange, Missouri. "I knew I had to quit, and not just for my
health. I could see that smoking was becoming socially unacceptable."

So in 1989, with some help from nicotine-laced chewing
gum, Kay gave up smoking for good. Gradually, she grew accustomed to a cigarette-free lifestyle; within 2 months, she
weaned herself from the gum. "I haven't craved a cigarette
since," she says. "If I'm someplace where people are smoking, I can hardly stand the smell!"

About the same time that Kay stopped lighting up, she

started cleaning up her diet. "I went through my cupboards and threw out all the snack foods, high-fat dairy products, and oils, except for olive oil," she says. She also replaced her reduced-fat milk with fat-free and changed her white bread to whole wheat. "Now I can't understand why some people prefer white bread," she says. "And if I drink any milk other than fat-free, I think it tastes funny."

In fact, Kay noticed that any time she made some adjustment in her diet or lifestyle, her tastes and preferences quickly caught up. "I never felt deprived, like I was missing something," she says. "Within a matter of weeks, I grew so used to each new habit that it seemed nothing had changed."

On the advice of her doctor, Kay was also taking Questran Light, a cholesterol-lowering medication. "It's a powder that I mix with fat-free milk and drink after each meal," Kay explains. Between that and her healthier lifestyle, Kay's total cholesterol dropped an amazing 100 points in just 8 weeks. It stayed around 200 until late 2000, when Kay's husband found out that he had type 2 (non-insulin-dependent) diabetes. "He had to give up refined sugar, so I did, too," she explains. "It was just like before: My tastebuds adjusted, and I hardly missed sweets."

Kay never expected that cutting out sugar would have a positive effect on her cholesterol reading. But it did. Her last test delivered the news she had been waiting for: Her total cholesterol had dropped to 170, with the ratio of total cholesterol to HDL cholesterol at a very healthy 3.6.

"Because my hypercholesterolemia is hereditary, I know I'll have to take Questran Light and stick with my lifestyle changes for the rest of my life," Kay says. "But I believe in preventive maintenance. These changes have given me a good feeling about my future."

· W I N N I N G   A C T I O N

Allow yourself time to adjust to new, healthy habits. Experts say that once you make a change in your lifestyle, you need at least 6 weeks to become acclimated to it. Be sure to give yourself that time. Gradually, the change will become second nature to you, and you'll all but forget about your old, unhealthy habit. Besides, once you achieve one change successfully, others will seem that much easier. Each one is a step toward a healthier cholesterol profile.

+++

FAMILY RALLIES
TO FATHER'S RECOVERY

Back in 1996, Mark Pagano thought he was in pretty good shape. That is, until he had a heart attack. He was only 40 years old.

A father of three, Mark had no family history of heart disease. He worked out regularly on a cross-country ski machine. In fact, he had dropped 30 pounds since 1993, leaving a trim 225 pounds on his 6-foot-4 frame.

So what went wrong? Mark places the blame squarely on his diet. "It was a mess," admits the human resources manager from Hummelstown, Pennsylvania. "I figured that if I worked out, I could eat whatever I wanted. I'd climb off my NordicTrack and help myself to a big bowl of ice cream." Just the year before his heart attack, his total cholesterol had risen to 262, which is considered high.

Mark's health crisis shook the Pagano family to its core. As he recovered, his wife, Eileen, became a driving force for change. "Like a lot of busy families, we lived on pizza and fast food," Mark says. "After my heart attack, Eileen decided that all of us were going to eat better. She went on a supermarket tour with a dietitian, she took low-fat cooking classes, and she converted a lot of our favorite recipes to low-fat. Finding ways to improve our eating habits became her passion."

Rather than ordering from a pizza place, Eileen makes a homemade version with low-fat cheese, or a stromboli stuffed with chicken and sun-dried tomatoes. In fact, chicken and turkey are popular dishes in the Pagano household. If the family eats ground beef, Eileen buys the leanest available.

Like eating healthfully, exercising regularly has become a family affair for the Paganos. On weekends, Mark and Eileen go to the local high school track for a 4- to 5-mile walk/run, often accompanied by their sons, ages 16, 13, and 10. Mark also visits a nearby gym three times a week, where he splits his hour-long aerobic workout between the stairclimber and the elliptical trainer.

Between his much-improved diet and his regular fitness routine (plus a daily 10-milligram dose of Zocor), Mark has kept his total cholesterol at a healthy level since 12 weeks after his heart attack. At one point, his cholesterol dropped so low—to 117—that his doctor told him to ease up on his eating habits. It has stayed between 150 and 165 since 1998. Mark's LDL is 87, his HDL is 49, and his triglycerides are 133.

As proud as Mark is of his improved cholesterol profile, he knows that much of the credit goes to his wife and sons. Their intervention and support enabled him to make the changes that were necessary to bring his cholesterol under control. "I always say that when I had a heart attack, my whole family had a heart attack," Mark observes. "All of us worked together to make our lives healthier."

W I N N I N G   A C T I O N

Turn cholesterol reduction into a family project. Whether you're working on improving your eating habits or establishing a regular exercise program, your immediate family can provide all the support you need to succeed. It helps to get them involved from the start, so they understand what you're doing and why. Who knows? They may decide to join you in your quest for a healthy cholesterol profile. Even if they don't have high cholesterol, the lifestyle strategies they'd be following can benefit them in other ways. Of course, just maintaining strong familial bonds is good therapy for a healthy heart.

++

HE FOUND A ROLE MODEL FOR SUCCESS

While attending the American Heart Association Scientific Sessions in 1986, cardiologist Peter Smith, M.D., of Galva, Illinois, discovered that his total cholesterol level was 245. He also discovered how bad some medical workers are at delivering bad news. "The technician who drew my blood told me that she was 'sorry for me,'" he says. "But I decided that this was not going to get me down."

Peter, who's now 47, had already gotten plenty of experience counseling patients on how to modify their risk factors to prevent progressive coronary artery disease. Suddenly, it was time to put that advice into practice for himself.

He started waking up a half-hour earlier so that he would have time to run before work. Before too long, he was running 5 to 7 days per week and up to 2½ miles per session. Even when he didn't run, he'd often spend time bicycling or cross-country skiing.

This may sound like a strenuous fitness regimen, but Peter

knew it was possible because he'd already seen it in practice while growing up. "My inspiration to start exercising comes from my father, who ran 5 to 7 days per week, 3 miles per day, from approximately 1950 through 1968," says Peter. "And he's continued to walk and ride a bike since then. At the age of 78, he rode his bicycle 5 miles up Going to the Sun Road in Glacier National Park."

In addition to the exercise, Peter adopted a low-cholesterol, low–saturated fat diet, and now he finds himself in the position of role model for the rest of his family. "My 16-year-old daughter works out on a NordicTrack ski exerciser every day and drinks only fat-free milk," he says. "My kids shun high-cholesterol snacks for the most part. My 6-year-old son comes downstairs at 10:00 P.M. and asks for his 'midnight snack'—a carrot. I think that my kids have gotten the message."

Peter has gotten a pretty good message himself. His most recent cholesterol readings include a total level of 196, an HDL level of 80, an LDL level of 103, and a triglyceride reading of 77. "The future is bright," he says.

WINNING ACTION

Find a healthy role model. It's often easier to adopt good health habits if you have someone else as your role model (or you want to be one yourself). Do your neighbors jog, ride bicycles, or play tennis? Suit up and ask if you can join them. Do you overhear coworkers talking about their weekend hikes or camping trips? Pump them for details of the experience and then invite them on a trip of your own doing. Sometimes, all it takes to get exercising is someone to talk to while you're doing it.

++

HE STARTED A CONTEST—
AND WON BETTER HEALTH

Before he entered college, Tim Rogers ran up to 18 miles a day. By the time he received his degree in 1993, he wasn't running anymore. His weight was up to 250, his total cholesterol was 256, and his LDL level stood at 193.

His weight continued to climb throughout the 1990s, forcing him to make several trips to the emergency room for breathing difficulties. "It seemed almost chronic that I'd get shortness of breath and feel light-headed," says Tim, who lives in Charlotte, North Carolina. His primary care physician kept telling him to lose weight and control his cholesterol, but Tim brushed aside the advice.

Finally, on January 5, 1998, Tim—by then carrying 294 pounds on his 6-foot-3 frame and still sporting a total cholesterol level above 250—decided to change his ways. What got him motivated? A New Year's contest with a friend to see who could lose the most weight in 2 months.

With the contest came a new approach to eating. Tim opted for pretzels instead of potato chips, used mustard in place of mayonnaise, ordered fish and chicken rather than beef, and cut out fried foods completely. "From January 5, 1998, to the middle of 1999, I didn't have a single french fry," he says.

As the pounds started coming off, Tim felt less motivated by the contest itself and more excited about the progress he had made. "At first, it was all about the weight," he says. "But you feel so much better after you lose some of the weight that it just becomes more a habit than anything else."

After a decade of inactivity, he finally began to run again. His wife, Michelle, kept him company while he ran, but they weren't exactly running together. "When I started running again in 1998, she'd lap me as I ran around the track," he says.

Nevertheless, he kept at his training and diet, and by July

1998, Tim's cholesterol numbers had improved dramatically. His total cholesterol had plunged more than 100 points to 152, and his LDL level was down to 96. What's more, by September, his weight was down to 195.

His friend dropped out of the contest, but Tim kept going. Before long, Tim and his wife were running side by side and even competing in marathons together. "It does help when you have other people trying to do the same thing," he says.

Still shunning mayonnaise and eating few fried foods, the 31-year-old now runs 30 miles a week to keep the cholesterol down and the weight off. The contest ended years ago, but he still feels like a winner at the end of each day.

WINNING ACTION

Start a friendly competition. If you have a friend or relative who is also trying to knock his or her cholesterol down, try to make a contest out of your efforts. Don't put too much emphasis on beating your opponent, though. The goal, of course, is for both of you to end up in the winner's circle, celebrating your victories for years to come.

++

EVERY DAY, HE WINS THE CHOLESTEROL WAR

Controlling cholesterol isn't a once-and-done deal. That's a lesson that 65-year-old Pascal Girard of Rehoboth Beach, Delaware, has learned from experience. Since undergoing open-heart surgery nearly 2 decades ago—when his total cholesterol hovered around 310—he's been working every day to keep his numbers in good shape.

After his surgery, Pascal adopted the Pritikin diet, practically the only cholesterol-lowering eating plan available at the time. "I cut out all simple sugars and refined flours," he says. "I limited my consumption of animal products, and I ate a lot of green vegetables. That took my cholesterol below 200 within a year."

Unfortunately, says Pascal, "I was doing so well that I also increased the meat in my diet—the lamb chops, the pork." In early 1995, after undergoing an angioplasty to correct one bypass, he switched to Dr. Dean Ornish's Program for Reversing Heart Disease—a combination of diet, exercise, and stress management—to keep his cholesterol low. He gave up meat, fish, and oils and returned to a nearly vegetarian diet. "That got my total cholesterol down to 157 in about 3 months," he says.

Then, early in 1996, despite a good total cholesterol level, Pascal's low HDL level of 35 became a concern. "I had been a heavy exerciser all my life," he says. "I was running 5 to 7 miles at a time, but only three times a week." He increased his workouts to six times a week, which boosted his HDL to between 55 and 60.

All along, Pascal's total cholesterol has been between 185 and 195. Keeping it in that range is an ongoing effort. "My wife and I went away for a week, and we ate out all the time," he says. "I gained 10 pounds, and my cholesterol probably went up, too." His neighbor was doing well on the Atkins diet, so Pascal tried it. He lost the weight, but his cholesterol spiked to 278.

Once again, it's on its way down, largely because of Pascal's continued commitment to his exercise regimen, his return to a Pritikin-based diet, and the addition of vitamin and mineral supplements to his program. He has cut back on running, instead spending time on the step machine at a local gym. His workouts are fueled by the compliments he receives from other gym patrons. "They tell me that I exercise twice as long as people half my age," he says. "I do the best I can."

W I N N I N G   A C T I O N

Acknowledge cholesterol control as a lifetime commitment. Lowering cholesterol isn't something you can cross off your to-do list, like other tasks and responsibilities. It requires constant awareness and vigilance, as every day can present new obstacles to eating well and exercising regularly. To keep yourself on track, consider posting reminders in locations where you're most likely to face decisions that could affect your cholesterol for better or for worse. Some suggestions: by the bread box, for when you're choosing between white bread and whole grain; on your computer, for when you might be tempted to eat a candy bar instead of a piece of fruit; on your sofa, for when you might be inclined to bag your workout and lie down for a nap. If you still slip up, don't despair—you have tomorrow to make it up to yourself!

+++

SHE ACHIEVED HER GOALS BY NOT SETTING ANY

April 1, 2000, was the day Linda Munson decided to stop fooling around and take control of her cholesterol by taking control of her weight. "I literally woke up one morning and decided, This is it!" says the 49-year-old resident of Sherburn, Minnesota.

Granted, Linda, who at the time carried 185 pounds on her 5-foot-4 frame, had tried to slim down several times before. And she had succeeded—but not permanently. The pounds always came back.

Then Linda bought a book that advocated a low-carbohydrate eating plan. She didn't try it right away, until she saw a friend who had lost a lot of weight on the same diet. That gave Linda the inspiration she needed.

Even when she committed to her new eating plan, she avoided setting specific targets for herself. "I'm not a person to set goals that require me to 'get those numbers down,'" she says. "It's too depressing if I don't reach those goals, and I tend to quit before anything positive is accomplished. Instead, I monitor my progress and am pleased with each step of the process."

By focusing on each positive step as it happened, Linda managed to lower both her weight and her cholesterol. Compared with readings from 1997, her total cholesterol level dropped more than 50 points to 228, her HDL level nearly doubled to 67, and her LDL level fell from 194 to 150. "Although the total cholesterol reading is still somewhat high, the change from the previous reading has impressed both my doctor and me," she says.

The rosier numbers should help Linda avoid the heart disease that has plagued her family, from a mother and father who underwent open-heart surgery to an uncle who had a heart transplant.

To continue her move toward a healthier lifestyle, Linda started an exercise program in October 2000 that consists of 30 minutes of aerobic exercise and 30 minutes of weight lifting four or five times per week. The exercise, combined with the low-carbohydrate diet, helped Linda drop 40 pounds in the first 5 months.

The lower numbers are great for showing off, but Linda says the biggest change is impossible to measure. "The positive feelings that I have about myself are the greatest reward for the effort," she says. "I feel better than I have in years and believe that I have a lifestyle I can maintain for the rest of my life."

WINNING ACTION

Focus on the process, not the goal. Sometimes when you set out for a distant goal, it's hard to tell whether you're

*making progress because the goal seems forever distant.
Instead of looking off to the horizon, focus on each step
that you're taking toward that goal. By knowing that
you're always moving ahead, you'll have the confidence
you need to keep going—no matter where the goal hap-
pens to lie.*

+++

HE'S MOTIVATED TO STAY AWAY
FROM DOCTORS

As a child, James Jochen had asthma. He grew out of it. But
even at the age of 75, his childhood experiences with doctors
and treatments color his life.

"I know what it is like not to feel well," he says. "I don't
want to have any association with the medical profession,
other than socially. I will do everything that's practical to
keep from being sick."

So when a general screening administered over 20 years
ago indicated that his cholesterol level, 235, was a bit high,
James and his wife, Gloria, changed their lives.

"We took most of the fat out of our diet," says James, who
lives in College Station, Texas. "We increased our consumption of raw vegetables. We increased our physical activity.
We knew what would happen if we continued to live the way
we were living."

While Gloria has mildly high cholesterol, she's not as religious about watching her diet. James, on the other hand, has
cut his red meat consumption "way down," concentrating instead on lots of fruits, grains, and nuts. He uses egg substitute, nonfat margarine, and low-fat alternatives to other foods
when they're available. "I take every opportunity to eliminate
fat," he says.

He has also cut back on sweets—"I haven't used sugar on
my oatmeal for years"—and walks 5 to 6 miles or bicycles

12 to 15 miles most days of the week. His cholesterol level now ranges from 150 to 175. His ratio (a comparison of total cholesterol to HDL), while varied, is always "proper," he says.

James and Gloria continue to work together in their healthy lifestyle. James gives Gloria full credit for her wonderful cooperation in providing food choices that fall in line with his chosen diet. "She does this for me, despite her lesser enthusiasm for the 'spartan' diets that I prefer, and that she has modified for herself," he says.

It's more than his dislike of medical treatments that motivates James. "I just want to live as long as I can," he says. "I have no intention of going, ever!"

And he believes that anyone with the same motivation can conquer cholesterol in the same way he has. "If you want to be healthy, you can do it."

WINNING ACTION

Be driven by a desire to remain healthy. Although we know that doctors strive to help their patients, some procedures they prescribe are uncomfortable or dangerous, not to mention expensive. Heart bypass surgery, for instance, is a serious operation and requires weeks or even months of recuperation. And cholesterol-lowering drugs, which experts recommend only after lifestyle changes have proven ineffective, are expensive and can cause side effects, including liver damage. As with so many things, prevention is worth more than the best cure.

++

HELPING OTHERS LET HIM
HELP HIMSELF

In 1996, Larry Walker had a heart attack. With a cholesterol level of 398 and a triglyceride level of almost 800, he knew that he had to take action. He went to cardiac rehabilitation, where he learned all about exercise, nutrition, and stress management. All was well until 1 year later, when Larry, now 53, had another heart attack. That time, he needed quadruple bypass surgery.

After a second stint in the cardiac rehab program, Larry, a resident of Midlothian, Virginia, started taking Lopid for his triglycerides and Lipitor for his cholesterol. He also joined the local gym, starting off with low-impact aerobics and working his way up to cardio kickboxing and Spinning.

The gym isn't all Larry joined. He also became a member of Mended Hearts, an organization affiliated with the American Heart Association (AHA) that's committed to helping heart disease patients, families, and caregivers. Eventually, the secretary of the local chapter retired, and Larry moved into that position. Soon, he was president.

As a member of the Mended Hearts organization, Larry visits heart patients in the hospital. That's given him the motivation to keep up with his healthy lifestyle. "Going to visit the patients reaffirms that I don't want to go through that again," he says. "And if I'm going to talk the talk, I need to walk the walk. I try to stay fit and upbeat and up-to-date on changes."

Being a part of this organization also keeps Larry educated on heart health. For example, in the spring of 2000, he attended an AHA meeting in Washington, D.C., where he heard researchers speak on advances in heart care. "The researchers seemed to think that if people with coronary artery disease can hang on for another 5 years, they'll probably have the cure," he says. "They'll change things like none of us ever dreamed." Larry also relearned information that he was too stressed to remember after his quadruple bypass surgery.

Larry's cholesterol level is now 99, and his triglycerides are 145. He has never felt better, and he partly credits the education he's received as a member of Mended Hearts. Says Larry, "It's empowering to realize that you can deal with heart disease and that you don't have to surrender to it."

WINNING ACTION

Join a health-related organization. Just belonging to such an organization will motivate you to make healthy lifestyle choices. Mended Hearts (www.mendedhearts.org) is one such group. To find others, try calling your local hospital or asking your doctor. Members of Mended Hearts receive the quarterly journal Heartbeat and have access to the "Members Only" area of the Mended Hearts Web site. Most important, members receive the support and encouragement they need.

++

HE GOT THE MESSAGE THAT HE COULD SUCCEED

Pedaling a stationary bike helped Marco Chierotti in his quest to lower his cholesterol, take off unwanted pounds, and regain his energy. But listening to audiotapes while on his bike instilled in him the motivation he needed to stick with his healthier lifestyle.

In the spring of 2000, Marco was ready to make some much-needed changes in his eating and exercise habits. By then, his cholesterol had reached 265—on top of a 30-pound weight gain over the previous 5 years. He was up to 232, more pounds than he needed on his 5-foot-10 frame. "I felt tired and blue. Life was not as good as it could have been," recalls the 40-year-old software programmer from Redmond, Washington. "I had no energy to exercise. In the morning, I'd need an hour just to roll out of bed and get ready for work."

His doctor's prognosis for a future riddled with health problems left Marco feeling even worse. Finally, he dragged himself to a local health club and signed up for a weight-loss program that had its own medical staff. Every week, he met with a dietitian, who coached him on food choices and dietary strategies. He kept a food diary, even documenting his fat and calorie intakes. He also met with a personal trainer, who set up an exercise program for him that included riding a stationary cycle.

When Marco's busy work schedule prevented him from attending the weekly support group meetings that were part of the weight-loss program, he was given audiotapes to listen to on his own time. He was also asked to attend some lectures on health and wellness.

The tapes, in particular, provided Marco with a wealth of practical advice that seemed to change his whole mindset. "They talked about ways to suppress cravings, to recognize emotional eating, to control portion sizes in restaurants," he says. "They even offered suggestions for organizing the refrigerator to prevent overeating."

For Marco, just as valuable as the advice was the sense of support that came from listening to the tapes, which he played during his cycling workouts. "The fact that the tapes were even discussing these matters made me realize that I'm not alone," he says. "They were proposing solutions and making sure I maintained a positive attitude, even when a lapse would occur."

The tapes convinced Marco that he should—and could—develop healthier habits. He gave up red meats, cookies, and ice cream in favor of chicken and poultry, green vegetables, and whole grains. He started running three times a week, in addition to stationary cycling and strength training.

In just 5 months, Marco successfully lowered his cholesterol by 72 points, to 193. He also shed 52 pounds, dropping to a much healthier 180. Perhaps as important, his attitude toward food is completely different. "Before, I would eat four or five cups of french fries and consider that a portion," says Marco, who's 41. "Now a portion is one cup. I used to love brownies; now I have no appetite for them. And I used to feel I couldn't leave food on my plate. Now I do it with ease."

WINNING ACTION

Listen to audiotapes for support and solutions. For cholesterol control, as for weight loss, educating yourself about your situation and your options is the first step toward success. An audiotape can be an ideal source of information as well as inspiration. It provides positive reinforcement for the healthy lifestyle you're trying to create. You should be able to find an appropriate audiotape in a bookstore or audio store.

++

SHE OVERHAULED HER LIFE— AND HER HEALTH

In 1998, Lucille MacNaughton and her husband, Fred, both newly retired, decided to break from their past and leave Glens Falls, New York. They ended up about as far away from their old home as possible: in Honolulu.

Right before the move, Lucille stopped smoking and took up cross-country skiing. Once in her sunny new home, the 56-year-old decided she needed to make still more changes. "I have three sons, and I've spent my entire life taking care of their needs," she says. "It's 'me' time now."

For Lucille, living in "me" time necessarily meant taking

better care of herself. "I was never physically active before moving here," she says. "I was pretty much overweight, close to 160 pounds, so I started walking a canal that I live on. It's 2 miles long, and I walked it every day."

Lucille continued this routine for more than a year. Then in April 2000, she developed hip pain that sent her to the doctor. There, she had her cholesterol tested for the first time. Even after a year of exercise and not smoking, her reading was an uncomfortably high 267.

Her doctor wanted to prescribe a cholesterol-lowering drug, but first, Lucille wanted to see what she could accomplish with more intensive lifestyle changes. She dropped meat and eggs from her diet, replacing them with fish and soy protein. For physical activity, she turned to water aerobics and swimming; later, she purchased a home gym. She also began taking a fish-oil supplement.

By September 2000, her total cholesterol level had fallen to 224, and her HDL level was an exceptionally healthy 74. "My doctor felt that if I continued to do well, medication wouldn't be necessary," she says. Actually, her doctor was so pleased with her progress that he decided not to check her cholesterol level again until another year had passed.

Today, the bulk of Lucille's diet consists of fresh fruit and vegetables, fish, and egg substitute. It's quite a change from her former eating habits, but she doesn't miss her old ways. In fact, she has created a whole new lifestyle since moving to Hawaii. In addition to taking art classes, Lucille—who now carries 135 pounds on her 5-foot-1 frame—is planning a bicycle tour of Europe within the next few years. "Coming here has been a radical, total life change," she says. "But it's been fun."

W I N N I N G   A C T I O N

*Put yourself in a different environment. Okay, so not every-
one can move to Hawaii, with its sunny days and endless
supply of fresh fruit. You can still change your surroundings.
Drop in on new restaurants in a quest for healthier dishes.
Visit the park to discover new walking and bike trails. Join a
bowling league or neighborhood association to cure
"couch potato-itis." The surest way to leave behind the
temptations of the past is to put some distance between
them and you, so start expanding your horizons today!*

++

NO KIDDING—SHE'S SLIMMER
AND HEALTHIER, TOO

When Joanne Moschella-Pearson started trying to lose
weight and lower her cholesterol, she had the entire city of
Pittsburgh watching her.

"In an essay contest sponsored by the *Pittsburgh Post-
Gazette*, I won a year of nutritional advice and fitness training with a personal trainer while the newspaper followed my
progress," says the 43-year-old stay-at-home mom. When
Joanne started her year's training in March 2000, she
weighed 199 pounds and had a total cholesterol level of 288,
an LDL level of 226, and a triglyceride reading of 116.

Once training began, the changes were immediate and dramatic. "I went from a virtual couch potato to someone who
put in 3 to 5 hours of 'target zone' cardio work and another
hour-plus of weight training every week," says Joanne. To
keep her pulse rate in a target zone of 142 to 170 beats per
minute, she bought a wireless pulse monitor to wear during
workouts.

"Finding the time to fit all of this in was a challenge at first
because I had two young boys in half-day kindergarten and pre-

school," says Joanne. "Babysitting arrangements were complicated, but after reading the newspaper articles, people started offering to watch the kids so I could get my workouts in!"

Joanne's children had also proved an obstacle in terms of her diet. "I'm always in the kitchen preparing meals, fixing snacks for the kids, or cleaning up," she says. To solve this problem, the nutritionist had Joanne log everything to do with her meals: the time of day, the quantity of food, how hungry she was before she ate, and how full she was afterward.

She also had to record whether the eating was "purposeful." "In other words, was I just grabbing a handful of snack crackers for myself while doling them out to the kids, which is not purposeful?" says Joanne. "I was surprised to realize how much food I actually ate without even thinking about it."

By October 2000, the 5-foot-5 Joanne had made great progress toward her initial goals, losing 15 pounds and dropping her total cholesterol level to 199, her LDL level to 139, and her triglycerides all the way to 55.

But the goals have become less important as time goes on. "This is a lifestyle now, not something I'll do just until I reach a goal," says Joanne. "I like having exercise be a part of my life, and I'm setting a good example for my kids."

WINNING ACTION

Hand the kids over to someone else and get out of the house. If you're a stay-at-home mom or dad, looking after your kids limits your exercise opportunities and encourages you to spend more time in the kitchen than you should. Hire a babysitter or ask a relative to watch over them a few times a week so you can make it out to the gym or onto the walking paths. If your kids are old enough, buy bikes or inline skates for everyone so that you can exercise together and set good habits for the future.

++

SHE'S MADE EATING RIGHT AND EXERCISING A LIFETIME HABIT

For her husband's evening meal, Margaret Hahn fixed him roast beef, gravy, and potatoes. While he enjoyed the fat-laden foods, she had green beans, fat-free cottage cheese with fruit, and a slice of whole wheat bread.

"I love to cook," says Margaret. "I bake a lot, and I enjoy doing it for my husband. He eats ice cream, steak, eggs, and regular margarine, and I eat my foods."

After 10 years, this has become her habit. But that doesn't mean that she isn't tempted every once in a while.

"I get upset with my husband for buying food when I can't eat it," she says. And sometimes she gives in. "But I feel very guilty when I eat anything I am not supposed to. I know what it'll do to me."

Margaret, who's 75 and lives in Ingleside, Texas, had high cholesterol—"quite a bit over 200"—the first time it was checked more than 30 years ago. Twelve years ago, when it soared to 303, she started working in earnest to get it down.

Now Margaret walks 3 miles every day and plays golf up to six times a week. "And I watch what I eat," she says. "I avoid red meat, butter, and cheese. I eat very few eggs, about two a week. I eat lots of fruits and vegetables."

She also takes the cholesterol-fighting drug Pravachol. Her cholesterol now measures 198, with an HDL of 48 and LDL under 125.

Margaret says that there is a history of strokes in her family. Her brother died at 56 after having a stroke a year earlier. "I enjoy life, and I want to have a good quality of life," Margaret says. "I just made up my mind that this is what I want to do."

Margaret says that sticking to her diet, even in the face of things like ice cream and gravy, is not difficult. Getting in a walk a day, despite the fact that her husband "goes around the block, then he drops off," is also not difficult.

"You have to get in the habit," she says. "You have to find out what the right things are to do, then just do them."

In 1995, Margaret was diagnosed with a clogged artery in her left leg. Doctors recommended surgery, but she refused, saying that she wanted to work on it through diet and exercise. While the clog is still there, she says, tests have indicated that her bloodflow is not impaired.

"This has gotten to be my lifestyle," she says. "I feel good, and I am enjoying life."

WINNING ACTION

Make eating right and exercising a habit. *Too often, we fall into bad habits: buttering potatoes when a touch of olive oil or a light sprinkling of Parmesan cheese works as well, eating ice cream every evening instead of a bowl of berries, reaching for a handful of cookies instead of a pretzel. But those habits are just that: habits. You can replace them with new, healthier ones. You just have to want to, and give yourself time to adjust to them. The same goes with your exercise routine. Start by building in small bouts of activity, like walking around the block, and build to bigger ones that you can live with for the rest of your life.*

++

HE SPREAD THE WORD ON HIS HEALTHY NEW LIFESTYLE

When Bob Perkins discovered the magical effect that exercise and a low-fat diet had on his health, he couldn't keep it to himself. So every morning at the restaurant where he has eaten breakfast for the last 16 years, he extolled the virtues of his newfound habits to friends and acquaintances who had noticed the healthy changes in him. By sharing his tips with others and showing everyone how well they were working for him, Bob was able to stay motivated himself.

All his life, Bob had been a "meat and potatoes kind of guy," consuming a steady diet of hamburgers, steak, and french fries. His idea of exercise was walking from his office to the car. When Bob retired in 1994, he became a flight instructor and later a pilot for an air ambulance company. "One day, we were loading a patient, and I began having trouble breathing," recalls Bob, who lives in Medford, Oregon. It turned out that he had coronary heart disease.

Despite medication, Bob's condition continued to worsen until he underwent emergency triple bypass surgery in 1996. Afterward, he was grounded by the Federal Aviation Administration because he didn't meet their medical standards. Determined to resume flying, Bob transformed his diet virtually overnight, with encouragement from his cardiologist and his wife, Jackie, a vegetarian. He gave up red meat completely, replacing it with chicken and fish. He also ate more fruits and vegetables.

With his flying career—and his life—at stake, Bob made changes beyond his diet. He began taking Lipitor and exercising fanatically. "My cardiologist, who's a fitness buff, said he wanted me at the gym every day, 7 days a week," Bob says. "In my mind, that meant it had to be better to go twice a day. My wife says it's called compulsive."

Spending so much time at the gym helped Bob lose weight quickly. His waistline shrank from 42 inches to 34 inches in 9 months. His friends at the restaurant where he ate breakfast couldn't help but notice the difference as Bob slimmed down from 230 pounds in 1996 to his current weight of 175. They also couldn't help but notice the drastic changes on his plate.

"I used to eat two eggs over easy, hash browns, sausage, and whole wheat toast with butter," he says. "Now I have oatmeal with brown sugar, raisins, and fat-free milk with a slice of sourdough toast dry."

What they couldn't see, Bob made sure to tell them. He

brought his stress test results to breakfast and gave steady reports on his cholesterol as it fell from a high of 222 when he had surgery to 105, his latest reading. Bob's subtle proselytizing worked. "Within months, some of my friends at breakfast changed their eating habits, and some even started going to the gym," he says. "One woman has lost 40 pounds. One guy has lost weight and now goes to the gym, too. He even has a personal trainer."

Bob says he didn't set out to tell people what to do, but he gets a good feeling watching others improve their health and likes prodding them on. He also knew that he had to stick with his new lifestyle if he was going to pontificate about it. "It's like going to a doctor who says you need to lose weight, and you look at him, and he's 80 pounds overweight," he says. "I felt I had to stay with it."

In 1999, Bob got the news he had been waiting for: The FAA lifted its ban and allowed him back in the cockpit. At 73, Bob knows he'll have to retire from flying in the next few years, but he's already contemplating his next career. "I'm kicking around the idea of speaking to groups on weight loss and cholesterol," he says. "I think it would be a lot of fun."

WINNING ACTION

Share your low-fat eating habits and exercise efforts with others. Talking to others about what you are doing will reinforce your commitment to a healthy lifestyle—and it may help encourage them to follow your lead. And if they join you, you'll find comfort in the camaraderie and joy in seeing others improve their health.

+++

BENCHMARK BOLSTERS
HIS FITNESS ROUTINE

At 4:45 almost every morning, Javed Rashid steps out into his still-sleeping Lahore, Pakistan, neighborhood for a walk. He sometimes gets lost in thought, but he never falls off his brisk pace. To ensure that he doesn't, he selects a benchmark—that is, he tries to cover a specific distance in a certain amount of time.

Javed, a 53-year-old electrical engineer, has been walking regularly since 1995, when he had a heart attack. His family gave him incentive to improve his health. "My children were very young, and I didn't want to put their futures at risk," he says. At the time, his total cholesterol hovered around 260, with an LDL of 192 and an HDL of 40. His triglycerides peaked around 400.

To improve those numbers, Javed set out to transform his eating habits. "The Pakistani diet is very poor," he explains. "Much of our food is high in fat and sugar. We eat a lot of meat, too." While the hospital had provided some nutrition information, Javed was more interested in Dr. Dean Ornish's Program for Reversing Heart Disease. He read about it in one of Dr. Ornish's books, which he had received from his brother—a doctor in the United States—about a month after his heart attack.

Javed styled his diet after the Ornish program, eliminating all meats and fish, dairy products, and added fats. For exercise, he had to find a substitute for running, which he was told he had to stop because of his heart. He took up walking, but even that was slow going at first. Right after his heart attack, he could walk for about 5 minutes before feeling fatigued. Over the next 6 months, he increased his workouts to about 45 minutes.

Next, Javed worked on accelerating his pace. His goal was to cover 5 kilometers (a little over 3 miles) in 45 minutes without significant discomfort. "I did this very cautiously, always mindful of the advice that if you can't talk while you're exercising, you're overdoing it," he says. "In about a year, I reached the benchmark I had set for myself."

Over the next 2 years, Javed was able to meet and sometimes even exceed his benchmark. Then he decided to lengthen his walks, in an attempt to get his total cholesterol below 210. Knee pain quickly put an end to his efforts. "I almost had to stop walking altogether," he says. "Now I'm very careful not to push myself so hard."

He doesn't need to. His latest test found his total cholesterol to be 166, with an LDL of 71 and an HDL of 42. His triglycerides have dropped by almost half, to 219. Though he takes a low dose of Lipitor, he attributes his successful cholesterol control to eating nutritiously and exercising regularly.

Now, Javed walks 6 days a week, usually covering his 5 kilometers in 45 minutes. He still aims for his benchmark in every workout, though it's so challenging that he attains it only about 60 percent of the time. That's okay. "The benchmark gives me something to work toward," Javed explains. "It encourages me to maintain my walking program."

WINNING ACTION

Set your exercise pace with a benchmark. If you're looking to liven up your fitness routine, or if you need help to maintain a consistent speed, consider designating a benchmark, as Javed did. If you walk, run, or cycle, it could be a certain spot on your route; if you strength train, it could be a specific amount of weight or number of reps. A benchmark gives you something to strive for. It may also encourage you to stick with your fitness routine. As Javed noticed, if he misses two workouts in a row, his performance suffers.

+++

AFTER THREE STRIKES,
HE'S BACK IN THE GAME

Fifty-five-year-old Michael D. Krebs Sr. took not one, not two, but three strikes before lowering his cholesterol. Luckily, life isn't a baseball game.

In September 1988, at the age of 42, Michael underwent bypass surgery on three arteries. He started taking Zocor and later Lipitor, which dropped his total cholesterol from a July 1989 high of 258 to below 200. But not much else changed in Michael's life. "I thought that because I had bypass surgery, everything would be hunky-dory," says this resident of Macungie, Pennsylvania. "I just did not take diet and exercise seriously."

Things were fine for 10 years. Then in early 1999, while having a stent installed in one of his bypass grafts, Michael had a mini stroke. He spent 2 months recuperating, which was ample time to finally start thinking more seriously about changing his lifestyle.

The final wake-up call came just 1 week after going back to work, when he returned to the hospital for a second stent installation. "During this procedure," says Michael, "my heart stopped, and I had to be 'zapped' while on the operating table." After his recovery, his neurologist recommended that he participate in a new education program on cholesterol, diet, cardiovascular disease, and diabetes (which Michael had developed in adulthood).

Since then, Michael has changed his life from top to bottom. He now walks 2 miles per day, five to seven times a week. He maintains a 2,000-calorie-a-day diet that allows a maximum of 35 grams of fat and 10 grams of saturated fat. He eats five to seven servings of vegetables and three to four of fruits daily as well as snacking on grape tomatoes and baby carrots. He eats more fish and poultry, particularly white meat turkey; he consumes no more than 6 ounces of red meat and two eggs per week; and he has significantly limited desserts, candies, and other snack food.

"There is no one thing—no silver bullet, so to speak—that an individual can embrace to miraculously reduce cholesterol," says Michael. "It requires several key elements of everyday living, blended together to help achieve the ultimate goal of cholesterol control."

But just because he's dropped his total cholesterol to 147 and lowered his weight from 232 to 183 pounds on his 5-foot-10 frame, don't assume that these changes always came easy for Michael. "It sometimes seems very unfair that so many people around me can enjoy so many things that I can't even begin to think of, let alone consume," he says. "Unfortunately, that's the way things must be—and that's what really constitutes a lifestyle change."

Overall, though, Michael has found that the good outweighs the bad. "Physically and emotionally, I feel better now than I have ever felt in my entire life," he says. "I have more energy, am more alert, and look better than I have since my early twenties. I know that what I am doing is the right thing and that I am prolonging my life by doing so."

WINNING ACTION

Approach cholesterol lowering as a total lifestyle change. Don't assume that dropping a single food from your diet or exercising once a week will bring your cholesterol level down. Examine your entire diet and exercise pattern and look for changes you can make in every aspect of your life. The more changes you can make, the more likely you are to put yourself on the path to good heart health.

++

OPTIMISM IS HER KEY
TO CHOLESTEROL CONTROL

First came high blood pressure, then high cholesterol, then diabetes, followed by hypothyroidism. But rather than wallow in self-pity about her health problems, Anita Goldberg thanked her lucky stars that she could do something to control them—and she does.

Anita, 57, of Springfield, Massachusetts, has had high cholesterol for 2 decades. She has hyperlipidemia type IV, a form of high cholesterol that is passed on in the genes. She also inherited high blood pressure from her mother and diabetes from her father. "Oh, yeah, I got the whole gene pool," she says.

On top of it all, Anita was overweight. In 1995, she tipped the scale at 152 pounds, more than she needed on her 5-foot-1¾-inch frame. Around the same time, she learned that she had type 2 diabetes. The normally optimistic Anita began to feel resentful.

"I'd say, 'Why is my body like this? I do all the right things, and my body isn't reacting the right way,'" says the nurse and grandmother of four. "But then I started thinking about other people, like my 44-year-old friend who died of non-Hodgkin's lymphoma. I decided that being miserable is a waste of energy."

Feeling empowered, Anita resolved to make changes in her diet that would help her control her diabetes. Those changes would ultimately help rein in her cholesterol levels, lower her weight, and enhance her feelings of control over her health and well-being.

Anita started following a doctor-prescribed liquid diet that included a small evening meal. For that meal, she limited starchy carbohydrates like bread and pasta, instead filling her plate with vegetables. When she ate salads, she doused them in red wine vinegar, lemon juice, or a combination of the two. Anita stayed on the liquid diet for 2 years. By then, her healthier way of eating had become permanently ingrained in her lifestyle.

In addition to eating better, Anita began walking on a treadmill three to five times a week, 30 minutes at a time. Her doctor prescribed several different weight-loss medications to help shed the extra pounds. She also tried different cholesterol-lowering drugs before settling on Lipitor.

Even a bout with hypothyroidism in the spring of 2000 was not enough to throw Anita off track, despite the weight gain it caused. With some help from medication, she was able to bring that under control, too, and shed 8 more pounds in the process.

No longer on thyroid medication, Anita continues to take Lipitor for her cholesterol, plus medicine for her high blood pressure. Her weight is down to 132 pounds—low enough to keep her in size-6 jeans. Her cholesterol, which used to be around 220, has now stabilized around 169. And her blood sugar is under control, too, thanks to the dietary changes she made.

"People get angry when their bodies don't do what they want them to," she says. "But if you have the power to impact your medical problem, you should be thrilled to death. There are people who can't and would love to trade places with you."

WINNING ACTION

Focus on what you can do about your health, not on what you can't. By dwelling on the positive steps you can take to change your condition, you'll be more likely to do so. Small successes will lead to bigger ones. You'll enjoy better health as well as the satisfaction of knowing that you are in charge of your own well-being.

++

A CLEAR MENTAL "BEFORE" PICTURE
WORKED WONDERS

Al Gentile remembers what he felt like before he started exercising. "I was moody," he said. "I'd get up in the morning and my pants didn't fit, and it would make me feel lousy."

That was before he lost 26 pounds. And now, when he needs motivation to get on the treadmill for his regular 60-minute workout, he just thinks back to those days.

"I like the way the exercise makes me feel," he says. "I'm not crabby all the time. You just have to tell yourself to do it."

Al, a 35-year-old Pittsburgh resident, started his weight-loss program as a challenge issued by the *Pittsburgh Post-Gazette* and the University of Pittsburgh Center of Exercise and Health Fitness Research. He and Joanne Moschella-Pearson, also of Pittsburgh, volunteered to be monitored for a year as they followed diets and exercise regimens prescribed by the medical center.

That was in March 2000. A year later, Al weighed 201 pounds, down from 227 (he is 5 feet 10½ inches tall). His cholesterol, only 197 to start with, dropped to 179. His HDL rose from 38 to 53, while his LDL fell from 138 to 112. And his triglycerides dropped from 103 to 73.

Al says that his diet only needed to be "tweaked a little." "We had to write down everything we put in our mouths for 3 days and then had an appointment with a dietitian," he says. "All she did with mine was adjust the portion sizes. I was eating a lot in great big portions."

But an exercise physiologist made a big change in Al's lifestyle. "I went from no exercise to exercise 5 days a week," he says. He bought a treadmill and worked up to 60 minutes a day at 4.3 miles per hour with the incline set on 4.5, which is equivalent to walking up a steep hill.

"If I don't exercise, I can definitely notice it," Al says. "I feel bloated, like I am full all the time, and I'm not light on my feet. I wish that I had done this before, but I was not raised in an exercise household."

Al says that the hardest part of an exercise regimen is finding the time to do it. He and his wife, Erica, have two children, 7 and 16 months. He is an engineer for GE Medical Systems.

"I have two windows of opportunity for exercise," he says. "One is early in the morning, like at 5:30 or 6:00. I'm not crazy about that one. The other is late in the evening, between 9:00 and 10:00."

He has a television set up in front of the treadmill, so that the 60 minutes goes quickly. "I feel much better," he says. "And exercise is what did it." That and the memory of those pants.

WINNING ACTION

Remember what your life was like before you changed it. Diet and exercise benefit us in so many ways, not the least of which is psychological. According to the U.S. Surgeon General's Report on Physical Activity and Health in 1996, inactive people are more likely to have symptoms of depression than more active people. When you feel good mentally, you're more apt to make other positive changes in your life. Of course, exercise is also a proven route to weight loss, which generally translates to lower cholesterol levels.

++

SHE ACTS NOW TO CREATE A BETTER TOMORROW

"Good things come to those who wait," the adage goes. But 33-year-old Scarlett Weakley Martin of Nashville, Tennessee, knows that sitting around won't do a thing for your high cholesterol.

By the time Scarlett graduated from college, one of her grandfathers had undergone bypass surgery, and her father had gone through two, including a quadruple bypass at age 40. Since then, her grandmother and great-aunt have had strokes, and her other grandfather has had bypass surgery as well. "It seems like it's just a matter of time," says Scarlett. "If you live long enough in my family, you get heart disease."

But she knew it didn't have to be that way. After taking a look at her total cholesterol level of 250, Scarlett decided it was time for a change. "I knew that I needed to eat healthier and fix the cholesterol problem, too," she says. "I realized that if I didn't start taking better care of myself, I could find myself in my father's position."

She started walking three or four times a week for 30 minutes to an hour, then moved up to running. "I thought I was too busy, but it was so important that I made it my top priority," says Scarlett, citing Stephen Covey's maxim: "Put the big rocks in the jar first." "You need to schedule the most important things, such as exercise, because the amount of time you need to do them isn't just going to pop up in your day!"

Her diet also went through dramatic changes. First came a switch to fat-free products, then the elimination of meat and dairy, and finally the introduction of whole grains. "You can learn to like foods that are healthy," says Scarlett. "It won't happen overnight, but exercising and eating right make me feel so much better that it's worth it for that alone, not to mention the future benefits. Life can hold a lot of joy even without a lot of deep-fried chicken and high-fat desserts."

Scarlett's total cholesterol level has stayed in the 190s for the past several years. With her family history, she doubts it will go lower. But with an LDL cholesterol level of 106, a triglyceride reading of 46, and a marvelous ratio (a comparison of total cholesterol to HDL) of 2.42:1, she feels good about the changes she's made, both for herself and for her family. "I plan to continue to take good care of myself," she says. "And now that I have a son, I have even more incentive as a role model for him."

WINNING ACTION

Do something to lower your cholesterol today, because tomorrow may be too late. You didn't build up a high cholesterol level overnight, so it's obviously going to take some time to lower your numbers to a healthy range. But instead of getting discouraged, use that knowledge to spur you to action. The sooner you get started toward your goal, the more likely you are to stay in the race and end up in the winner's circle.

++

RESOURCES

✦ ✦ ✦

40 FOODS THAT CAN MAKE
OR BREAK HIGH CHOLESTEROL

Of all the factors that can influence your cholesterol level, diet may matter most. After all, any cholesterol your body doesn't make on its own comes from foods, especially animal products. They're high in saturated fat, which raises the amount of LDL ("bad" cholesterol) circulating in your bloodstream.

But not all foods send your cholesterol skyward. Those with good amounts of fiber can help lower cholesterol by escorting any excess from the body. And foods well-endowed with antioxidants such as vitamins C and E and beta-carotene keep LDL from oxidizing, so it doesn't harden and clog arteries.

The following chart lists 20 foods that can help you win the cholesterol war and 20 that can prolong the battle. While these lists aren't exhaustive, they can point you toward dietary changes that will support your efforts to control your cholesterol and protect your heart.

+++

FOODS TO ENJOY

Food	Portion	Fiber (g)	Vitamin C (mg)	Vitamin E (IU)	Beta-Carotene (IU)
Apple	1 medium	3.7	8	0.7	42
Apricots, fresh	3	2.5	11	1.4	1,662
Blackberries	1 cup	7.6	30	1.5	144
Black currants	1 cup	8.2	202	0.2	156
Broccoli, cooked	½ cup	2.3	62	2	684
Brussels sprouts	½ cup	2	48	1	336
Butternut squash	½ cup	3.4	18	0.2	5,124
Cantaloupe, cubed	1 cup	1.2	68	0.4	3,096
Carrot	1 medium	2.2	7	0.5	12,150
Chickpeas, cooked	½ cup	6.2	1	0.4	12
Green peas	½ cup	4.4	11	0.2	288
Papaya	½ medium	2.8	94	2.5	255
Passionfruit	5 medium	9.5	25	1.5	390

Food	Portion	Fiber (g)	Vitamin C (mg)	Vitamin E (IU)	Beta-Carotene (IU)
Raspberries	1 cup	8.4	31	0.8	96
Red bell peppers, chopped	½ cup	1.5	31	0.8	1,482
Red grapefruit	½ medium	1.4	42	0.5	90
Spinach, cooked	½ cup	2.2	9	1.3	4,422
Strawberries	1 cup	3.8	94	0.3	24
Sweet potato	1 small	3.4	28	0.5	14,922
Wheat germ	¼ cup	3.7	1	3	—

FOODS TO AVOID

Food	Portion	Saturated Fat (g)	Total Fat (g)	Calories
Bacon double cheeseburger	1	19	39	640
Baked potato with cheese sauce	1	11	29	475
Barbecued ribs	3 oz	9	26	337
Beef hot dog	1	7	16	180
Butter	1 Tbsp	8	12	110
Candy bar, chunky	1	8	10	170

Food	Portion	Saturated Fat (g)	Total Fat (g)	Calories
Cheddar cheese	1 oz	6	9	115
Cheesecake, homemade	1/12 of 9" cake	18	33	455
Chocolate mousse, homemade	1/2 cup	19	33	445
Coconut cream pie	1/8 of 9" pie	10	17	260
Cream cheese	2 Tbsp	7	10	100
Doughnut, cream-filled	1	6	21	305
Fried chicken	2 drumsticks, 1 thigh	10	37	624
Hot wings	6	8	33	470
Ice cream, premium	1/2 cup	11	18	270
Pork sausage, smoked	3 oz	10	28	345
Prime rib	3 oz	13	31	355
Ricotta, whole-milk	1/2 cup	10	16	216
Sausage biscuit with egg	1	10	28	440
Taco salad, with shell	1	14	52	850

INDEX

✦ ✦ ✦

Underscored page references indicate boxed text.